MIND MEDICINE FOR PAIN RELIEF, STRESS, AND ANXIETY

MINDFULNESS PRACTICES USING THE INNATE ABILITY OF YOUR SUBCONSCIOUS MIND, BREATHWORK, AND MEDITATION TO FIND HEALING AND PEACE IN YOUR LIFE

DR. JORDAN BURNS

© **Copyright 2023 - All rights reserved.**

The content contained within this book may not be reproduced, duplicated or transmitted without direct written permission from the author or the publisher.

Under no circumstances will any blame or legal responsibility be held against the publisher, or author, for any damages, reparation, or monetary loss due to the information contained within this book, either directly or indirectly.

Legal Notice:

This book is copyright protected. It is only for personal use. You cannot amend, distribute, sell, use, quote or paraphrase any part, or the content within this book, without the consent of the author or publisher.

Disclaimer Notice:

Please note the information contained within this document is for educational and entertainment purposes only. All effort has been executed to present accurate, up to date, reliable, complete information. No warranties of any kind are declared or implied. Readers acknowledge that the author is not engaged in the rendering of legal, financial, medical or professional advice. The content within this book has been derived from various sources. Please consult a licensed professional before attempting any techniques outlined in this book.

By reading this document, the reader agrees that under no circumstances is the author responsible for any losses, direct or indirect, that are incurred as a result of the use of the information contained within this document, including, but not limited to, errors, omissions, or inaccuracies.

CONTENTS

Introduction — 11

1. MINDFULNESS — 15
   What Is Mindfulness? — 15
   Types of Mindfulness Practices — 17
   Benefits of Mindfulness — 28
   Tips for Practicing Mindfulness — 31
   Action Step — 34

2. THE SUBCONSCIOUS MIND — 37
   What Is the Subconscious Mind? — 37
   Parts of the Subconscious Mind — 39
   Metacognition — 41
   Healing Using the Power of Our Thoughts — 46
   Daily Habits — 54
   What We Give Energy to, We Give Life To — 59
   God-Given Medicine (Healing from the Universal Intelligence) — 62
   Action Step — 67

3. THE EGO — 69
   Is Ego Really the Enemy? — 69
   Disadvantages of the Ego — 74
   The Five Steps of Ego-Work — 76
   Action Step — 80

4. STOICISM — 81
   What Are You Afraid Of? — 81
   A Brief History of Stoicism — 82
   Memento Mori — 86
   Death and Mortality — 87
   How Do You Want to Be Remembered? — 88
   Trauma and Life Struggle — 89

After Accepting Your Fears	92
Action Step	96

5. CREATIVE VISUALIZATION — 99
- Can You See It Healed? — 99
- Creative Visualization for Pain Relief — 101
- Creative Visualization for Stress and Anxiety — 104
- Action Step — 106

6. GRATITUDE — 109
- What Are You Grateful For Today? — 109
- Best Ways to Practice It Daily — 111
- Practicing Gratitude for Pain Relief — 113
- Practicing Gratitude for Stress and Anxiety — 115
- My Take on Gratitude — 116
- Action Step — 117

7. POSITIVE AFFIRMATIONS — 119
- Who Do You Want To Be? — 119
- How to Use Positive Affirmations — 120
- How Can Positive Affirmations Be Used for Pain Relief? — 123
- How Can Positive Affirmations Be Used for Stress and Anxiety? — 124
- Action Step — 126

8. MOVEMENT — 127
- How Can You Prioritize More Movement? — 127
- Benefits of Exercise for Pain Relief — 129
- Benefits of Exercise for Stress and Anxiety — 130
- Walking Outside — 131
- Action Step — 134

9. BREATHWORK — 135
- Can You Visualize Your Breath? — 135
- Benefits — 138
- Can Breathwork be Used for Pain Relief? — 139
- Can Breathwork be Used for Stress and Anxiety? — 140
- Best Breathwork Techniques for Beginners — 142

	Personal Notes	144
	Action Step	146
10.	MEDITATION	147
	Is Meditation the Key to Peace?	147
	Stress, Anxiety, and Meditation	149
	Elements of Meditation	149
	Meditation and Pain Relief	151
	Personal Take on Meditation	151
	Benefits of Meditation	152
	Action step	153
	Conclusion	155
	References	157

To my beautiful wife, Kayla

You are, without a doubt, the greatest thing that has ever happened to me. You are what I prayed for. I am a better man because you are in my life. You are the truest, kindest person that I know and you inspire me to be the very best version of myself.

"Watch your thoughts. They become your words. Watch your words. They become your actions. Watch your actions. They become your habits. Watch your habits. They become your character. Watch your character. It becomes your destiny."
–Lao Tzu

INTRODUCTION

In this book, you will learn about how mindfulness can positively impact your health, happiness, and overall quality of life. The purpose of this book is to show you how the thoughts you have (Chapters 2 through 5), the words you use (Chapters 6 and 7), and the actions that you take (Chapters 8 through 10) can reduce your levels of pain, anxiety, and stress. Using the techniques and concepts in these chapters, you'll be able to bring a healthier and happier version of yourself into being. The information isn't overly technical or super complex—the purpose is for anyone and everyone to be able to use the powerful tools that are their thoughts, words, and actions to improve their life.

I want to share a story to put this all into perspective. I once had a patient who had cancer for more than two years and was in extreme pain every day. The pain medication had stopped working; the only thing remaining to manage the pain was to get onto morphine. She didn't want to do this because she felt like morphine was a hard drug that would lead to rampant addiction (especially considering she'd never taken hard drugs in her 54 years). So, she decided to start a new regimen in addition to taking her pain meds. She started practicing grounding, positive affirmations, walking for extended periods every day and began a highly nutritious diet incorporating multiple homemade juices daily. With this routine she created, she could keep herself off morphine for a further year (while in stage four) because the pain had become manageable.

Like my patient, you might have aches, pains, body difficulties, anxieties, stress overload, or other things you want to control in your body and mind. You might want to avoid going down a route relying expressly on pharmacology. Or, you might feel it's not severe enough yet to call for an intervention, but this condition is proving to be a continuous source of annoyance. In this book, you will learn various techniques to use your mind and body to accomplish healing and personal elevation. By learning and using these techniques, you'll bring your health and happiness under your control, thus, keeping your well-being in the hands of someone you know you can trust—you.

The information you'll learn in this book comes from someone extremely passionate about natural health and wellness and the use of the subconscious mind to uplift your life. I hold four college degrees (a Bachelor's in Kinesiology, a Bachelor's in Life Sciences, a Master's in Sports Science and Rehabilitation, and a Doctorate in Chiropractic). Over my seven years in practice, I have also developed a love for personal development and philosophy. Holistic health gives me unending enthusiasm because I love when people can alleviate pain, stress, and anxiety by gaining calmness, stillness, and peace. As a believer, husband, father, and just a man that cares about the health of humanity, knowing that I can provide my family, friends, and community with ways to heal themselves naturally provides me with immense satisfaction. Let's get started.

1

MINDFULNESS

"If you want to conquer the anxiety of life, live in the moment, live in the breath."

— AMIT RAY

WHAT IS MINDFULNESS?

Before we get into how our thoughts, words, and actions can be used to help us heal naturally, I want to explain mindfulness and provide a plethora of examples of how to use mindfulness in your everyday life. Mindfulness is being in the present moment rather than thinking of the past or plans for the future. It also refers to the practices associated with improving or maintaining your ability to be in said state. However, it's more than just being in the present. It also refers to being present while being aware of yourself and what's happening around you.

In terms of yourself, mindfulness includes awareness of what's happening within your body and your mind. Externally, the state consists of awareness of where we are and what's happening in our vicinity. This awareness is continuous and follows from one moment to the next, always being in the present (in other words, it can be called systematic awareness of the present, where we are in the present, and what's happening around us). Practicing this awareness makes us much more capable of bringing our attention back to the present when it drifts. It requires acceptance of where we are and what's happening in and around us.

Mindfulness is associated with our ability to process information. The information we're processing is in the present or relates to what we're doing now and helps to cut out a lot of noise, allowing us to focus far better on the task at hand. As such, we release thoughts or thought patterns that continually disturb us, freeing our minds to process things that need our attention for the work we're busy doing.

A few notes about mindfulness:

- Not judging ourselves is an integral part of mindfulness and mindfulness exercises. We need to

accept how we exist and what we think. Only after we've faced our reality and the reality around us will we have a starting point from which to operate.
- Mindfulness can become a habit that forms a part of a more stable and easier-to-live life. Our mind doesn't splatter everywhere with a resultant state of feeling overwhelmed. It's us becoming more settled with ourselves and our lives.
- Mindfulness doesn't change who we are. Instead, it brings out who we already are so that our innate personality shines. Our present self stands out with ourselves extricated from the press of future desires and past pains or experiences.

TYPES OF MINDFULNESS PRACTICES

We increase our level of mindfulness by using practices that have been used and developed for this purpose. Some of these techniques are thousands of years old, stretching back to Ancient Buddhist practice. Others are modern developments.

Mindfulness Meditation

Meditation is the most well-known mindfulness practice. There's a whole host of meditation techniques you can use, including ones you can do while lying down, sitting, standing, or even moving. Loving-kindness meditation is one of the core meditative techniques to improve mindfulness. It's a meditation technique that we use to enhance compassion for others and ourselves.

Overall, mindfulness meditation is when you use meditative techniques to slow down and separate yourself from the hubbub of day-to-day living. It's about centering yourself so that you can focus on the things that affect you on a deeper level and so that you can put the fleeting thoughts in your mind to sleep for mental clarity. You bring yourself to "now" and focus on the present world. You raise your awareness of your body, its sensations, and its position—paying particular attention to breathing deep and slow.

It isn't something that needs to take you hours and hours; you can do a few minutes of mindfulness meditation when you have the time available. In all honesty, while a quiet and distraction-free environment is best, you can still do a mindfulness meditation session in a relatively busy area where you know you won't be bothered for a few minutes.

While you do this, you will have thoughts demanding your attention, but this is your time to disengage from all that. Acknowledge the thought and bring your attention lightly back to your breathing. After a few minutes, you'll notice that you don't feel as "scrambled" and that you're in a better mindset to confront the demands of the day once again.

Mindful Movement

Mindful movement is a catch-all phrase for mindfulness practices that incorporate movement. Some of these practices include movement meditation, yoga, and qigong. Movement meditation is where you go through actions deliberately and slowly, using all your senses to notice what's happening. This type of meditation doesn't require you to sit still, nor does it require taking time from your day to go through different poses. All you need to do is be mindful of your body as you're doing what you're doing (like noticing your breath, feeling the pressure of your feet against the floor, and feeling your heartbeat).

Yoga is a practice that involves moving through different poses to strengthen your body and mind. The purpose of yoga exercises has traditionally been to increase self-awareness, particularly on a spiritual level. Practicing yoga while using mindfulness increases its benefits. Breath awareness, observing the sensations and pains in your body while holding poses, and observing the things happening around you. Observe without judging what's happening (i.e., not forming opinions or decisions about it) or reacting to what's happening internally or externally. Just be there and experience the moment and the poses. If you have wandering thoughts, gently acknowledge the thought, then bring your attention back to the present.

Qigong is a type of martial art. The purpose of qigong is to strengthen your body and balance out your energy. Meditative qigong is about relaxing your mind and body. The movement patterns are often done slowly, focusing your attention on what you're doing and making sure you take long, slow breaths. Tai chi is one of the best types of qigong, which can also be done for mindfulness purposes if you have the correct types of motions, stretches, and stances.

Journaling

Journaling is something that you can easily do at any time, anywhere. All you need is something to write with and some paper to write on. It's a good way of getting the things floating around in our heads into the real world. Many mindfulness practitioners suggest using free association when journaling, as this allows you to understand your mind better. Free association is when you let your thoughts flow one after another, even if there's no apparent connection between one and the next. It gives you a greater understanding of yourself, especially subconsciously.

It's been shown that journaling reduces stress as well as anxiety (Smyth et al., 2018). Other proven benefits include reduced mental distress, a heightened level of resilience, coping with trauma or grief, and a lower incidence of pain affecting your daily activities. Many of the things you'll write are fleeting thoughts or thoughts that you usually only vaguely consider. As such, you won't only acknowledge the thoughts and let them out of your mind, but you'll also solidify them on paper, thereby getting to know yourself better.

It would help if you had a judgment-free mindset when writing down your thoughts. You won't be able to grow personally and build a mindful perspective if you're censoring your thoughts and not confronting their reality. This exercise aims to clarify ideas that come and go and approach your daily thinking with a curious mindset. In many cases, you gain new perspectives that allow you to see the world differently. The way to do this to get the best results is to express yourself fearlessly. Share your feelings, whether good or bad—contentment, stress, anxiety, boredom, excitement, you name it. Write whatever comes up, and if you notice you're veering off track, bring yourself back with a few minutes of focused breathing before you continue journaling.

A related exercise you can do is expressive writing. In this exercise, you write about a traumatic experience or an experience with many emotions tied into it. Write about it for 15 to 20 minutes every day for four days. This practice helps process through feelings and stray thoughts connected with the experience, freeing you from complicated emotions or at least helping you face those emotions and thoughts head-on. Writing about it might make you feel negative emotions and not enjoy the exercise fully (although many people do appreciate it). Yet, some benefits make the activity worth it. Benefits include long-term physical health benefits (such as your lungs functioning better) and emotional health benefits (such as a lower incidence of avoiding traumatic events after they've happened) (Baikie & Wilhelm, 2018). Of course, you'll also be able to experience life more mindfully because blockages will hold a less potent grip on your mind.

Body Scanning

This is a very straightforward exercise. You focus on successive parts of your body (usually from the top down or bottom up, but only sometimes). A lot of the time, imagining the body part you've got your attention on will help, especially when you're not yet able to directly sense that body part. If you can perceive the senses relevant to that part of the body, pick up what you can. Besides increasing mindfulness, this exercise aims to improve our sensory experiences.

Body scanning is often done to alleviate pressure, pain, or discomfort in a particular body part. This can be done by using breathing while you meditate. Breathe in while visualizing calm energy and relaxation coming into your body and flowing to the part that isn't feeling as it should. Then breathe out while visualizing the pressure, pain, or discomfort released from that part of the body. You can do this on one part of your body, or you can do it on multiple parts of your body. It's also advisable to do this as a repeated practice to get maximum benefits.

Progressive muscle relaxation is a similar practice to reduce unwanted sensations in your body and calm your mind. You do this by tensing muscles in your body, then relaxing them. If you tighten your muscles, the sensation of relaxation is more pronounced afterward, emphasizing a physical perception of ease in your body. The muscles systems should be addressed one after another from head to toe and back up to your head. Your mind gets the opportunity to unwind as your body feels calmer. This is an excellent exercise to carry out while lying down before trying to get some rest.

Grounding

You can do grounding (also called earthing) every day to connect yourself to the world while improving your health. You can do it to start your day by standing barefoot on the grass while you take five or more deep belly breaths. After I take my breaths, I say prayers for my family, friends, community, the world, and me. By doing this, I simultaneously connect myself to the Earth's surface electrons, Mother Nature and God.

I started using grounding a few years ago when I had a change of perspective about how I saw humanity. I visualized everyone as their nervous systems. I imagined the brain, spinal cord, and peripheral nerve roots for every person on the planet—their complete nervous system with its interconnection between all the muscles, organs, and tissues of their bodies. I realized that everyone is essentially an extension of the "Earth's nervous system."

Nobel Prize winner, Richard Feynman, explained what I realized in lectures about electromagnetism. He said the body's potential and Earth's electric potential are the same, resulting in grounding. The body, thus, becomes an extension of the Earth's electric system. These lectures are why I am so passionate about my job and grounding. When I can help improve the connection between the brain and the body, the connection between the body and the Earth is even better.

The research that's being done on grounding shows that having contact with the Earth can be a potent way to combat chronic stress, pain, inflammation, lousy sleep, autonomic dysfunction, and other health disorders. It's a simple solution that can have profound effects. Coupling this with nutritious meals, physical activity, clean water, sunshine, and fresh air is how we can stay healthy naturally.

Visualization

Visualization is when you picture things in your mind to bring them into existence. Some visualization practices can increase our mindfulness, while others are used for different purposes (such as actualizing our goals). Color breathing is a practice to increase mindfulness, wherein you decide on something you want to bring into yourself (such as confidence). You then assign it a color (such as purple) and breathe in. The trick is to imagine the air you're breathing in as purple (i.e., the color you've assigned to confidence). Visualize yourself breathing out junk and unwanted things with each breath, making a place for more purple to saturate your body. Visualize your entire body becoming saturated with that color.

Guided imagery is another effective visualization technique to increase your mindset. It works by relaxing your body through exposure to pleasant ideas. When your attention is on unpleasant thoughts or ideas (such as something you're scared will happen or something that just happened that you're angry about), your body tenses up. Likewise, when you think of something pleasant (such as a calm waterfall or a place where you had a good family holiday), your body relaxes because your mind has calmed down.

What you need to get started is some time in a quiet place where you'll feel reasonably comfortable. It's helpful to read through a guided imagery script or two at some point before attempting it so you can visualize the joyous scenes you can imagine. Some people enjoy doing guided imagery along with an audio recording where there's an instructor calmly guiding you along as you have your session. You can use apps to do this, such as Calm, where you can access other features, such as setting up a daily visualization and meditation routine.

Mindful Breathing

This is done by controlling your breathing. The purpose is to lower stress and increase awareness of the air going in and out of your body. Feel the sensation of the air entering and leaving your body. Sense the expansion and contraction of your lungs and diaphragm. Strictly speaking, mindful breathing doesn't require altering how you breathe. All it needs is that you're wise about how you're breathing, bringing you back into the present moment and reducing your stress levels.

Exercises can be done where you alter your breathing, breathe in a specific way, or do particular tasks while focusing on your breathing. These breathing exercises can also be used to increase mindfulness and reduce stress, despite not falling into the strict definition of mindful breathing. The most common breathing exercise used to grow mindfulness is to breathe in slowly, holding your breath for a few seconds, and then breathing out. This can be repeated a few times. The benefit of this exercise is that you have a sudden rush of oxygen entering your system, which in turn causes your body to function more calmly and reduces the stress or anxiety you're feeling at the moment.

Deep breathing exercises can also be done to immense benefit. Mindfulness is incorporated into these exercises because your focus is naturally brought to the present when you focus on the motion of air in and out of your body. With deep breathing, you force your breathing to slow by ensuring that you inhale as much air as you comfortably can and then exhale fully. The process involves focusing on the expansion of your lungs while your diaphragm contracts and then the shrinking of your lungs as you exhale and your diaphragm relaxes.

Sensory Exercising

Exercising your senses makes you wiser. At the same time, exercising your senses is good for increasing mindfulness when you mindfully do them. In other words, when you use your senses to perceive things happening in the present, you're conducting a mindfulness activity. This can be done with anything you're busy doing. For example, if you're walking outside, use your senses to heighten the experience and become more mindful. Smell the trees and grass, feel the sensations of the wind and clothes on your skin, and so forth. You'll notice there's a lot more to what you're doing than just walking outside–it's a whole experience.

Improving your sensory perception increases the amount of information you have when making decisions. You have information coming from multiple perceptive organs, and the information, once integrated, provides a complete picture for you to work from. When, for example, you're looking at someone you want to work with, and you notice their eyes are shifty, and you hear there's a quiver in their voice, then you know that it might not be the best idea to rush into things because there's something they're nervous about or that they're hiding. If you're in your own world and need to be mindful of your conversation and not using your senses to the level you can, then you'll miss social cues like this at work. You'll save yourself a lot of future stress, confusion, and sleepless nights if you increase your mindful use of your sensory organs.

Pausing

You can take a pause at any time of the day when things are just becoming too hectic, and you need them to slow down for a moment. It's calming and can bring our emotions back under our control. Stop what you're doing for a few seconds or minutes and close your eyes. Breathe in and out, putting your attention on your body and physical sensations. It can be helpful to repeat a favorite mantra or affirmation to yourself before opening your eyes again.

BENEFITS OF MINDFULNESS

Mindfulness has a ton of mental and physical benefits. Being mindful of the things you're doing results in you completing your tasks at a higher level of quality and a higher rate. Besides the other benefits we'll cover in this section, getting your daily tasks completed faster and better is a blessing in and of itself. The stress levels melting away as you meet deadlines and fulfill obligations makes the time and attention you dedicate to mindfulness worth it. This is mainly due to the increased focus you can dedicate to the work you need to do and the sustained periods at which you can maintain those levels of focus.

The physical symptoms that arise when you're going through a lot of stress are reduced when you're conducting your day with mindfulness. The stress reduction means that your body doesn't need to be as tense (in case you need to handle arising emergencies and demands) as when you're being less mindful. Your muscle tension should release somewhat, and the frequency of headaches (particularly pressure headaches) should decrease. If you get digestive problems because of the nerves you've built up, relaxing with mindfulness should ease these complaints. Reducing these physical symptoms of stress will also have short and long-term health benefits. Also, raising your awareness of your body reduces obsessiveness about health symptoms (i.e., hypochondria) because you're more aware of the good and bad things actually taking place in your body.

When you're being mindful, other conditions relating to your effect should lower in intensity. This includes depression and symptoms related to depression. When you have depression, being mindful can ground you in the present and disengage you from the sources of your depression in many cases. Controlling your emotions should also be more manageable. This is because you react less to emotional triggers if your attention is in the present rather than the past. And when negative emotions do rise to the surface, such as when you're having a heated discussion with someone, you should be able to tolerate them better because you're grounded in the present, and your effect has an overall calm to it.

The calmness of your effect should also positively impact your mental functioning (like processing of information). You're taking in a lot of information because your attention is on the various information sources around you. There's less rumination of that information because your mind is occupied with the things you're busy facing right now. This increases the level of clarity with which you see things and improves the data quality of your working memory. Many people who practice mindfulness find they're also less likely to lose track of what they're doing, even if there are multiple trains of thought and numerous tasks they need to keep track of in a given time period.

Grounding yourself in the here and now makes it easier to keep track of yourself better. You've improved your awareness of your body functions, and you've reduced the levels of mental clutter by remaining mindful. Thus, it gets easier to look at your own mind without becoming distracted or overwhelmed by a multitude of experiences. Being more aware of yourself and improving your self-control has a definitive positive effect on your well-being. It's easier to accept yourself as you are because you have to face fewer things about yourself at once. With acceptance, it also becomes easier to be kind to yourself because there are fewer instances of feeling overwhelmed and like you're being inadequate in relation to the tasks you need to get done.

Being calmer about who you are and where you are allows you to set your direction more easily. With your focus on the task at hand, you can steer your actions more diligently toward the goals you've set for yourself. This is particularly true because distractions will take up less of your time and energy, freeing up more "mental resources" to dedicate yourself to the actions that advance your personal targets. You'll further gain a more complete perspective of your life because you'll better understand where you are now in relation to the goals you've set for the various aspects of your life.

It's easier to keep an external perspective in mind when you're observing the things happening around you and when you're more at ease with yourself. This allows you to increase the attention you have available to place on others and the things they're doing or saying. When you're observing how someone's doing as they're communicating with you, then your reactions can be more appropriate (i.e., your emotional intelligence goes up). The result is that your relationships with others will improve in quality, and you won't come across as indifferent. People will perceive you as more compassionate, and they'll be able to share important information with you more comfortably.

Increased attention on others is instrumental in relationships with our intimate others. Our person relies on us for emotional support and to provide a non-reactive environment for them to talk about the things that frustrate them or challenge them. If we understand their communication better and respond more appropriately, there will be less reason for interpersonal conflict to arise. And if a conversation does lead to conflict, you'll be able to return to a baseline of serenity faster once the argument is concluded. As such, the relationship becomes healthier, and a more supportive environment is created in the home.

TIPS FOR PRACTICING MINDFULNESS

Doing visualization meditation might be easier to do before delving into other forms of meditation with the purpose of mindfulness. For those with a lot of thoughts going on simultaneously, it might be easier to focus on images you're creating in your mind rather than working towards clearing your mind of extraneous thoughts. It's also particularly for people who don't find it easy to contact their inner world (i.e., their feelings, thoughts, values, etc.). When you can't reach your inner world easily, using your imagination first can be an excellent way to break down the walls blocking that self-contact.

Putting a time limit on your session is something you can do to ensure you stay calm when you start. If you've done a few minutes and feel better, don't force yourself to delve into more profound thoughts, emotions, and experiences until you're ready. Another way to make it easier for yourself when you're starting out with mindfulness exercises is to make sure you set up a daily routine that includes some time for mindfulness. It's far easier to gain the benefits of mindfulness when you do it routinely, and there is little time between sessions, or the sessions occur sporadically.

Have something to put your focus on when you're practicing mindfulness. This could be music in the background, an object in our vicinity (when you're practicing with your eyes open), or your breathing. Having something to focus on can ground you when your mind becomes busy. But if you do lose focus while being mindful, don't criticize yourself too much. Take note of what distracted you (i.e., what thought or area of thought took your attention), acknowledge that it happened, and lightly bring yourself back to being mindful.

Mindfulness doesn't only have to be practiced in a mindfulness session. Use it in your daily activities. If you're going to wash the dishes, feel the water's temperature and smell the dishwashing liquid as you're busy. Bring your attention to what you're doing as you're doing it. You'll find that it makes your daily living much more comfortable and less stressful because you get a lot more done, and you find the things you get done more interesting. As a suggestion, get some mindfulness time scheduled into your working days because your work will often be the thing that takes up most of your time while you're awake, and it will often place the most demands on you. Having some time for mindfulness at work every day (even if only a few minutes) will raise your productivity and make your work more rewarding on a personal level.

In a workplace setting, you might even find a few of your colleagues would be willing to try out some mindfulness, especially if you show them some of the productivity increase stats that have been published showing the results of mindfulness. In this case, you can even do a mindfulness group session as part of the day's routine. You and the colleagues meet up. You check in about each other's state mentally, physically, and emotionally (without getting too deep into it). Then you all close your eyes and focus on your breathing for a few minutes, perhaps with some light music in the background or a guided meditation playing from someone's phone or computer. After a few minutes, everyone opens their eyes again and briefly describes how they feel after the session. Repeating this daily can provide a significant boost to the team.

In terms of your mindset while doing mindfulness practices, I'd suggest keeping a sense of curiosity. When you're curious about what's happening, you innately have an interest in what's going on. Further, there is a low level of judgment because you're examining rather than deciding what to label the things or actions you're observing. Keeping yourself in a relaxed, curious frame of mind goes a long way forward.

ACTION STEP

Do a mindfulness session with yourself today. Take ten minutes and find a quiet space, whether in your room, outside or in an empty office. Check-in to see how you're doing physically and emotionally. Take note of how you feel, but try to avoid over-examining or introspecting too much. Take a few deep breaths to infuse your blood with oxygen and to activate your parasympathetic nervous system. Close your eyes and use your senses to notice what's happening in the surrounding environment. Also, use your internal senses to feel what's happening in your body. Do this for a few minutes. Each time your mind wanders away from gently noticing what's happening in your body and your environment, acknowledge the thing that pulled your attention away, then bring your attention back to the mindfulness session. Once a few minutes have passed, open your eyes and check in with yourself about how you feel now physically, mentally, and emotionally. Your session is now finished, and you can resume your daily activities.

2

THE SUBCONSCIOUS MIND

> "Whatever your conscious mind assumes and believes to be true, your subconscious mind will accept and bring to pass. Believe in good fortune, divine guidance, right action, and all the blessings of life."
>
> — JOSEPH MURPHY

WHAT IS THE SUBCONSCIOUS MIND?

Our thoughts create our reality. Before you can genuinely understand this concept, you need to have a good understanding of what the subconscious mind is and how it works. Your subconscious is the part of your mind that operates beneath your awareness level. It conducts more than 90% of your mental functioning (Molitor, 2019). It stores your memories, influences your choices, relates your current experiences to your past experiences, and influences your general effect. Without realizing it, our subconscious is always aware of what's happening in and around us. It's constantly exerting its influence on the things we do and how we do them—always having its grip on us beneath our awareness.

Despite its constant influence, the subconscious mind isn't immune to our influence. We also have a say in what happens. In fact, we have more authority over what goes on in our lives than our subconscious; we just need to know how to operate it properly. When you don't know how to manage it, your subconscious processes unchecked and does whatever it sees fit. Oftentimes, this leads to misguided conduct and occasionally to negative emotional states. Reprogramming our subconscious is the first step in recuperating from this.

When you reprogram your subconscious, you get it to do what you want it to do. You take charge of it and use it as a tool to advance the things you want in life. The effect of doing this is increased happiness, a more accurate display of your personality and wants, and a healthier you. Who you are will affect what you do, and when you reprogram your subconscious mind, you'll express who you are in a more authentic fashion. You'll be able to take what you go through daily as a lesson that contributes to personal growth rather than a trigger to a subconscious reaction.

You'll see your subconscious mind express itself in your dreams, in the way you represent your artistic sense, and in the things you say "without thinking." When you've identified it better by knowing what to look for, you'll see its effects more and more. You'll see how it makes you anxious and alters your behavior in ways that don't align with your intentions. You'll also see the good effects it has due to the positive inputs it uses. This includes things like the way you bring across your creative expression and the way you do things without thinking (such as making tea).

One of the more essential functions of the subconscious mind is to bring the body and mind back to homeostasis (i.e., a state of equilibrium). Your body functioning (such as your heartbeat and your breathing) is governed by this. The temperature of your body and its chemical reactions are also under its control. Without your subconscious mind, you would have to focus on all these things as they happen (which would be impossible considering the sheer quantity of things happening in your body at any given moment).

PARTS OF THE SUBCONSCIOUS MIND

Your subconscious mind is constructed from multiple components. The memory bank is one of the main components. They contain the most complete storage of personal experiences in your mind. Most of the things you've lived through are recorded in minute detail, so even if you can't remember something while thinking of it in the present, it doesn't mean you don't have that memory. The storage banks have a near-infinite amount of space for all the future memories you will record. Their purpose is to guide you along with your future actions by leaning on the learned experiences of past actions.

The senses are part of the subconscious mind. When you pick up information through your sensory channels, your subconscious captures the information. It then determines the quality of the information and gives feedback to the conscious mind about what was observed. Further, it instructs the body and conscious mind to feel what the senses have shown should be felt (like feeling a blade and instructing the body that it should feel sharpness and pain). You can then use this information to make decisions about what to do and about what's happening.

There's also the storage for the routines you use in your life. Routines include the repetitive actions you do without really thinking about it (such as tying your shoelaces). Habits are also recorded in this part of the mind. The habits you have that you do without even noticing (such as always desiring and getting chocolate when you're sad) are stored here. There is also storage in this part of the mind for language capability. The routine recognition of words, symbols, and sounds gets ingrained here so that you can communicate freely with others without having to consciously think about how to speak, listen, read, or write.

The final part of the subconscious mind creates thoughts. The thoughts generated can be conscious and lead to thinking by the conscious mind. It can also generate unconscious thoughts that are beneath the awareness of your conscious mind. The information gathered to develop these thoughts comes from the other three parts of the unconscious mind (the memory banks, the sensory part, and the part that deals with routines).

Your personality is also influenced by your subconscious. This is because it holds a lot of control over your past experiences and what you use those experiences for (in terms of behavior). It's also because your subconscious mind affects the way your sympathetic and parasympathetic nervous systems operate, as well as how your mind processes new information entering it. As such, your motivations, level of confidence, general demeanor, and positivity are all influenced by your subconscious.

METACOGNITION

Metacognition relates to our ability to regulate our thinking and learning. It can be defined as "thinking about your thoughts" (Chick, 2013). In other words, when we observe the processes that happen in our mind and we're aware of why we're carrying out those processes, we're using metacognition. It further includes monitoring our level of understanding about the things we learn and observe, as well as the amount of learning we've done on a particular subject. This makes metacognition a quantitative and qualitative action, albeit the action leans slightly towards a qualitative nature.

There's a critical aspect to metacognition. You're not simply observing the things you're learning but also making evaluations about how you learned and how good your learning ability was in relation to the information being gathered. Further, metacognition includes critical observation of your thinking as separate from learning. In other words, the thoughts you're thinking of at any point of the day can be evaluated by you in terms of their origin point, the processes used to develop them, and the accuracy of those thoughts— this is metacognition.

The level of your metacognition skills is classifiable into four degrees (Perkins, 1992). At the bottom rung, there is tacit metacognition, which is where you don't have an awareness of the processes that are taking place in your thinking (i.e., you're thinking without knowing how). The next step is aware metacognition, where a person knows what processes are taking place in their mind (or at least some of the processes), but the person has no influence on those processes. The third level is strategic metacognition, which is the further step wherein you use the mental processes to forward your intentions. The final step, reflective metacognition, is when you not only organize your thinking processes toward your goals but also notice when those processes aren't happening up to the standard needed, so you alter them accordingly.

In other words, this final level is where students can observe how they think and learn as they do those activities and make appropriate adjustments for maximum success.

This top level of metacognitive skill contains two main elements—monitoring and controlling. Monitoring is where you can observe your mental processes as they take place (i.e., strategic metacognition). Monitoring is vital to proper learning because without it, you won't know whether you understand the information presented to you. The information will just be there, and if you don't understand it, you'll blissfully continue learning with no idea that you're confused or not fully grasping something. The second element, control, is where you adjust the processes you're using to rectify misunderstandings. Examples of this are when you replay a part of a video you're learning from or when you Google the definition of a term you don't understand.

These two main elements are of importance because you have the power to improve them. You can practice your ability to monitor your thinking or your learning. This can be done by going through questionnaires after you've studied some material or by asking others whether your understanding is the same as theirs. Honing your monitoring abilities will make you an acute self-observer so that you can track your comprehension of inputs. Controlling can be practiced by stopping yourself when your monitoring has shown you're not fully grasping information. Study up on different ways you can clarify confusions, misunderstandings, and incomplete ideas while learning. You'll likely get descriptions about tools like rereading a piece of information, clarifying with your instructor or the person you're having a conversation with, and searching for more information online, amongst others. Practice these tools so that you can fill in the gaps as you learn. The pace of your learning is less important at first, but rather the level of your understanding.

There are further steps you can take to improve your metacognitive skills. These can be broken down into different levels of assessment. One assessment should be done before you try to learn something or try to think about something in a different way. This assessment requires that you look at how you're thinking or how you're thinking about a subject before trying to learn or make changes. The next is to assess when you need clarification while learning something. Note the points that you need help figuring out so that you heighten your awareness of information not fitting in with other information. You will need this skill so that you don't apply incorrect information or incorrect understandings to situations in your life.

The following assessment is an assessment once you've completed learning or making changes to your way of thinking. This will allow you to see how your overall grasp and any changes that you successfully made to your knowledge base or cognitive processes. If you notice changes, validate them by acknowledging that they took place. A final assessment is to track your thinking processes on a continuous basis with the purpose of raising your awareness of how your mind works. This is done by keeping journals of the way you think, the conclusions you draw, and the information you use to make decisions. The journal (or alternative such as a daily checklist where you check in with your mental activities for the day) should be used until you feel you're comfortably aware of your thinking. Also, how you control thinking, where you fail to control it, and where you have room for further improvement. You must understand how your thoughts flow to learn at your best level.

As part of your self-assessments, you should note your strengths and weaknesses. By noting where you're weak, you'll see where you need to improve. But, perhaps just as importantly, you need to see what your strengths are. You're going to use your strengths to advance in life and to organize your life into your vision, with the added benefit of reducing your stress. This will only be possible when you know what skills (on a mental level) you have operating at the highest level and can thus take the most advantage of. When you see your strengths, acknowledge them and use them. If you're a good listener, for example, then you know that you'll be able to learn well by attending lectures, listening to audiobooks, and watching videos. Likewise, when you know you're a good listener, then you'll be good at handling a lot of social demands and actually coming to a mutual understanding with the person who's talking. If this is the case, it would be beneficial to use your skill (listening) extensively in your working and personal life (such as going into customer support or becoming the family mediator and thereby creating a less stressful home life).

Take control of your thinking by doing this. You'll thank yourself for it. It's not just your conscious mind that will benefit, but your subconscious too. Your subconscious is where you gain sensory information, relate information to past experiences, and use habits. By using metacognition, you can make sure that the sensory messages you gathered are correct; the experiences will be less likely to influence you in unintelligible ways because your subconscious mind will see when there's clearly no link between a memory and input you've just gathered. Your habits can be altered into ones more conducive to success because you're consciously altering them by repetitively refining them or changing them.

HEALING USING THE POWER OF OUR THOUGHTS

Your thoughts aren't set in stone. You are their master and can dictate what your mind should be doing. We use this ability to utilize the power of the mind to meet the demands of our lives. The abilities of the mind to sense, learn, organize, plan, and think are what make us stand out as the dominant species on the planet. But, our mind doesn't have to be limited to handling the demands placed on us in our work and personal bodies. It can also be used to heal our bodies.

The way you speak to yourself and the way you think affects your outlook on life, as well as the functioning of your body. Your body will respond as if it's in a dangerous situation if you're scared about something that might happen. In this case, your blood will flow to your limbs so that you can confront threats or flee from them. Your heart rate will go up, and your breathing will hasten. If you're constantly in fear, other reactions can include migraines, muscle pain, and breathing difficulties, amongst others. Thus, someone who is going through a really tough time in their life, such as doing an internship with a terrible boss who constantly threatens to fire them, will start having some of these symptoms due to their constant fear-related thoughts and reactions.

In the above example, the thoughts and physical reactions are largely the results of the subconscious mind's functions. It's not only the conscious mind that affects our biological functions and health, but also the subconscious. In fact, it's mainly the subconscious mind that you have to thank for the emotional state and resultant bodily reactions. The subconscious mind sends you signals that the input from your environment shows that you're in a dangerous situation and that you should fear potentialities because there have been negative experiences in the past that have similarities to what you're currently going through. It, thus, instructs your body to react accordingly in an effort to prevent negative eventualities, and it alters your emotional state so that you're hyper-vigilant of further threats in your environment.

Your immune system is also affected by your mental state. When you're stressed or depressed, your immune system functioning changes (Dispatch Health, 2019). This means that you're more prone to getting ill when you're under negative stress or when you've been driven into a depression. Conditions that can be brought about by depression include heart problems, autoimmune illnesses, and infections. Stress causes a cornucopia of negative health conditions, including exacerbating asthma, gastrointestinal issues, obesity, and heart problems (Griffin, 2014).

The solutions that you can use easily to alter your thinking so that you reduce your risk of exposure to those conditions include the direct methods of hypnotherapy and conditioning, along with indirect means wherein you make changes in your environment.

Hypnotherapy is where you see a professional who can guide you into a trance-like state wherein you can easily focus inwards. It's easier for you to review yourself in relation to your personality, behaviors, motivations, habits, etc. With the help of a professional, you can make changes you desire to make when you're focusing inwards in this state. The changes can have permanent positive changes in your life, whether it be because of how you look at life or because of the ways you think and act. When doing hypnotherapy for a while, your internal awareness and control will increase to the point where you can more easily make the changes you desire by yourself (i.e., without guidance from a hypnosis professional).

In terms of your physical health, hypnotherapy-induced changes can bring your mind into a state wherein you're not unnecessarily using negative trains of thought or operating with an undesirable effect. As such, you only perceive stressful situations when there is real stress, not when there's a non-stressful situation that reminds you of a past interval of stress. Thus, your immune system will not be under undue pressure, resulting in lower performance.

Conditioning is where you induce a reaction to a particular stimulus by repetitively introducing that stimulus and requiring an action as a result of the stimuli, often followed by a reward or pain depending on the action that was done. An example of this is when people of previous generations were spanked when they swore. As a result of multiple instances of pain induced by spanking along with a reprimand, people of those generations generally didn't swear when confronted with situations that frustrated them (the situations being the stimuli). Using rewards can be seen in situations where a person in the workplace is provided with recognition, gifts, or other desirables (such as a day off) when they achieve high levels of performance. The reward provided to the employee serves as motivation to continue acting with high-performance levels when provided with quotas or targets (the stimuli).

You can introduce conditioning as a control to alter your thought patterns to a healthier level. The idea is that you change the neural pathways that your mind has established to perform thoughts and actions habitually. These pathways form a routine for you to perform the same action with little to no resistance. This is because you don't have to put much input into it (i.e., you don't need to waste your time and energy to work out how you're going to do something each time you do it). This is particularly useful when you're stressed and can only dedicate a little energy to figuring out new ways of doing things you've done in the past. To change the way you think, you'll need to utilize neuroplasticity by introducing a new way to do something or think about something.

Introducing this new approach can be done in multiple ways, with writing down what you want to have, do, or happen being one of the most effective ways. You'll need to repetitively practice these new approaches or ways of thinking so that they become the mind's go-to process, action, or thought pattern to utilize in relevant contexts. In doing this, the old neural pathways become less used than the new ones, and your behavior changes permanently. One example is when you write down your daily to-do list using positive rather than negative language, such as "I'm completing..." rather than "Don't forget to...." In doing this, you're shifting your focus to what you're doing rather than the stressors or penalties that wait if you don't do it. This healthier mindset will calm you down and, in the long run, will eradicate multiple stress-induced health issues.

There are other direct means of altering thought patterns, but these are mainly covered in other parts of the book. They include things like meditation and guided imagery. On the flip side of the coming, we have indirect means of thought change. Indirect means to alter your thoughts are to change the environmental cues that cause you to use unwanted thought patterns. When these triggers relate to stress, the practice is called stress management. The simplicity of it is that you're going to find what causes you to feel stressed (or to feel a different negative emotion), and you're going to find the things that make you think in unwanted ways, then you're going to remove them from your environment, or you're going to remove yourself from their environment. This isn't always possible, but in many cases, you would be surprised to see that you can remove those triggers or, at the very least, reduce their presence in your life.

An example of how this can be done is when you note that one of the main things that stresses you during the day is seeing a colleague that's threatened you in the past. A simple step you can take is to change where you sit in the office so they're not constantly in your peripheral vision. If you get a seat that faces in the opposite direction, you're not looking at them all the time. You might still hear them when they're talking or see them when you or they are walking around the office, but there will be a drastic reduction of their presence in the attention you have available to give. With your mind not constantly taking note of their presence and bringing up the memory of their threat subconsciously, you'll find yourself feeling slightly less stressed, and you'll have more focus on the work at hand.

Self-care is a necessary undercurrent for indirect thought-change measures that you're implementing. The care you give your body and mind makes it easier for you to readjust to a calmer state. Getting good sleep is one of the steps to take here. When your body has the energy it needs from rest, you won't be constantly fatigued, and you'll be able to focus better on what you're doing. When you don't sleep enough on a regular basis, your body will be induced to produce more adrenaline, thereby triggering your fight or flight response and putting you in survival mode. This counteracts the stress reduction changes you're making. Other self-care steps to include in your daily life are eating healthier meals in the right quantities and having time each day to yourself to unwind.

The result of changing your thinking is that your body will be more at ease, and there will be more opportunities for your brain to release dopamine and serotonin. As such, it'll be easier for you to experience joy and to be motivated. You'll enjoy your interactions more and feel less anxiety and discomfort. With your body functioning more regularly and less in survival mode, your health will be positively affected. Over the long term, this will mean your body will be less predisposed to infections and diseases—even some chronic conditions.

The Placebo Effect

The placebo effect is where you have a reaction to medicine or similar substances, even though you weren't actually given the medicine that you thought you'd taken. In drug studies, this happens when you're in the control group (the group that wasn't given the drug but rather a fake), yet you still have a reaction. There are a few explanations for this reaction, both mental and external. The cognitive explanations are that you had an expectation that something positive was going to take place, so your body or brain complied. Another mental reason is that your mind had attention on the "cure" in question, so there was less attention on the condition or pain. Conditioning is also a mental explanation for the placebo effect. Your body will react accordingly when you've been conditioned to believe that you feel better or you're getting better because you took medication. This is also true if you think you were part of a healing practice. Then the body will react according to the automatic responses it's been taught (i.e., exhibiting certain positive symptoms).

One of the external explanations is that you were provided with care. When you're provided with care (such as being checked up on, being cleaned when you can't do it yourself, and being fed with nutritious food), then you're going to have improvements in many conditions. Even when the treatment you've received is fake, high-quality care will have positive mental and physical effects. Social support will also give you a boost because you're being enticed into a positive mindset or being shown that there are beings that value you. Stress reduction will also benefit you when undergoing treatment because you're not in the presence of all the stressors you face daily. Even when you're just staying home rather than in a facility, you're still removed from the environments where you work and socialize, thereby cutting out any stressors or triggers those environments induce.

The placebo effect shows us that the mind and your thoughts have a powerful impact on your body's healing. While there are non-mental aspects to the placebo effect in some instances, it's clear that many people have improved their health based on mental perceptions and changes. Your mind has healing powers. You are far more powerful than you currently think.

DAILY HABITS

I often tell patients that "the hardest habit is doing the easy habits consistently every single day." Your habits are contained in your subconscious, and they're established with the purpose of making it easier for you to do the things you need to do. With established habits, you don't have to waste any of your valuable attention. This means that habits are definitely helpful to you, especially if they're healthy habits. If you have habits that aren't healthy or desirable, they can become a stubborn thorn in your side. Your mind has already made them an integral part of your everyday functioning on a subconscious level, so there are multiple things you're going to have to do to disestablish them or to establish replacement habits. The habits you might have problems with can affect you mentally, physically, emotionally, or spiritually. When you've deleted them from your life, you'll find there are fewer barriers for you to overcome.

The first step to altering or eradicating a habit is to be aware of it. This will require introspection, particularly since much of the habit will be beneath the level of your conscious mind. To become aware of it, take note of your environment, the physical sensations you experience, your emotions, and your current thoughts. This will give you a holistic view of yourself and your relationship to the environment around you. When you've already been using mindfulness techniques for a while, this will be far easier because you will have a higher quality of observation skills. Metacognitive skills that have been practiced will also come into use because you'll have learned how to observe yourself strategically and to spot incongruities easily in your thoughts, behaviors, and your learning.

When you're aware of the habit you're trying to bring to a conscious level, you can see what it consists of. You'll notice what areas it affects in your life, what triggers the habit, and the actions or thoughts you carry out when the pattern is in effect. Eradicating the trigger for the habit or reducing its presence in your life should be the follow-up step. If you have a problem with wasting time on lunch breaks, you might see that the trigger for this habit is that you don't like speaking with the person at the reception desk because they're overly chatty. Seeing that this is the case, you could alter your lunchtime so that you're scheduled to come back when that receptionist is on their break.

You'll need to come up with a behavioral alteration that you can use in place of the habit. In the case of the receptionist, the pattern to overcome is avoidance of chatty people. To introduce a new practice will require a conscious attempt at introducing a new routine for you to use in place of the old one (i.e., you're setting up a new neural pathway). Once you've worked out the new routine you'd like to establish, it will require repetitive use of the routine until it's established itself. This should be broken down into steps so that you can repeatedly add new parts to the habit before adding a whole new habit.

So, when you have trouble handling conversations with chatty people, for instance, an excellent way to introduce a new habit is to attend a communication course. The course can provide you with theory and practice to understand the steps to take when handling conversations with people who talk excessively. With the steps practiced, you can start applying the skill in real life and establish communication habits that make it easier for you to handle such interchanges. At this point, it will no longer be necessary for you to use your altered lunchtime, so you can revert to your original lunch break because it will be easy for you to smoothly end your conversation with the receptionist without being rude.

Reprogramming your subconscious mind will require more work than altering a habit, although it will follow a similar process. You'll need to ensure that you've done a lot of self-awareness skill-building. You need to understand your subconscious thoughts, beliefs, and habits. Your thoughts generate your beliefs and habits, so it's helpful to know what your thoughts consist of and lead you to conclude. Once you've established an overview of what goes on in your subconscious mind, you know what parts of it you want to change and what parts of it are operating as you want it to.

When you've determined what the state of your subconscious is, you can establish goals and targets about where you want it to be. Your targets will determine how you want to think, how you would like to behave in general, and what beliefs you would like to have to underlie your conscious thoughts. The purpose of establishing goals is to know the destination that you're trying to reach from the perspective of your current reality. The tool to do this is to establish the change you want consistently.

As with altering habits, changing your subconscious is only possible when you repeat the changes you want to establish. So, in terms of thoughts, you need to use tools such as using affirmations and looking at quotes from people you would like to be like regularly. You will be able to alter your mindset by doing this over and over and over. You can do this in a targeted way. To do it in a targeted manner, look at the types of thoughts you would like to change specifically. If you have a lot of sexual thoughts, and you want to think less sexually, then it will be of use to affirm the things you would like to think about—i.e., don't affirm "I'm thinking less about sex," but rather "I'm thinking about a healthy relationship." If you use the former, then you're inevitably going to try to force yourself not to think about sex, which in turn will do precisely the opposite because you're giving the subject of sex your energy. But, if you focus on thoughts about healthy relationships, then you're dedicating your mental energy towards exactly that. In the end, you're going to find yourself thinking more about different ways you can establish and solidify mutual support in your relationship.

Your beliefs and your habits will naturally alter with the change in your thinking. The beliefs and habits rest upon the thoughts you have, after all. The fact that you've changed the way you think will mean that you've disengaged from past types of thinking, which in turn means that you'll have disengaged from past habits and forms of behavior that are incongruent with your new way of thinking. As a result, your past experiences have a lower influence on you in terms of being stimuli for negative behavior because your consciously ingrained habits and thought processes have seniority to those that were naturally established by the subconscious without your direct input. You should have lower levels of fear, anxiety, and doubt as a result since you're there's less indirect influence from the past. The fear, anxiety, and doubts you have should have more validity because they're based on present-time evaluations of present risks and observations without undue influence from irrelevant experiences.

Following through with the above steps will ally your inner world and behavior with the state of being you intend to have and convey. As Leon Ho (n.d.) states, "Your subconscious mind is a field, your thought is a seed, and the fruits you produce are habits (good or bad)."

WHAT WE GIVE ENERGY TO, WE GIVE LIFE TO

The thoughts you have exert an influence on the subconscious mind. It's not a one-way relationship of the subconscious continually influencing your behavior and thinking. There's give and take. The things you think can have as much influence on the subconscious as the things observed in the external world, sometimes more. As your health, happiness, and quality of life are influenced so heavily by the subconscious mind, it's high time you provide it with the fuel it needs to contribute rather than detract from the reality you would like to create. This is done by dedicating your energy to thoughts, subjects, and acts relevant to the personal reality you would like to exemplify. For instance, if you want to be a socialite with large-scale influence, then you've got to start thinking about all the people you're contacting and all the campaigns you're reaching out to. You need to think about these things instead of the distance you have between your current social media following and your desired one. Otherwise, you're going to be dedicating energy to the fact that you don't have enough people in your following.

When you're not meeting the expectations you have in life, it's okay to be upset, frustrated, or dissatisfied. But you can't go into a state of self-pity where you overanalyze your perceived inadequacies. If you do this, you're just going to emphasize the weaknesses in your daily behavior. Yet, if you focus on the goals you've set, there will be a higher likelihood that you bounce back and do the things you want to. You're dedicating your energy to what you want to achieve, so your subconscious continually brings its attention to the goal you have in mind. It will use the habits, routines, and information available to advance that goal because you've indirectly instructed it that you care more about the goal than the failure.

Due to the importance of dedicating your energy to your goals, the goals you set should be of high quality. To do this, establish noble goals. A noble goal is a high-level goal that encompasses an overall contribution you would like to make to the world. In other words, it is the change you would like to affect with what you do. It guides all your conduct because it's the constant underlying motivation for the things you do. Other goals link, thereby aligning multiple activities towards the same overarching intention. Suppose your noble goal regarding your work is that you would like to make a more ethical business environment. In that case, your other goals and resultant behavior will align toward creating a more ethical environment. A more ethical environment is accomplished by influencing your subconscious and conscious minds with the energy you've put into the goal (particularly when you repeatedly affirm this goal to yourself to maintain its relevance every day).

Noble goals guide your conscious decisions every day. They don't take problems the external world throws at you into account because they're above those barriers. The goals are oriented in an outward fashion because they are relevant to the changes you want to bring about. Since they're externally oriented, they guide you to exert your influence. As such, you're less under the influence of victim mentality because you know you're bringing about changes in the world around you. Thus, a noble goal serves to inspire you, no matter the challenges you face. (Note that I'm not saying there isn't such a thing as a victim, and I'm not saying that victims aren't entitled to redress for the wrongs done to them; I'm stating that you'll feel less like a victim and there will be a reduction in any sense of helplessness).

One of the best things about a noble goal is that it has durability. Its endurance is due to it going beyond the daily struggle. It's a profoundly rooted goal that adjusts your habits and neural pathways to align with it. The durability of the goal means that it provides an endless source of motivation. You might have short intervals where you're down, but they don't align with the energy you're directing to the change you want to make, so rebound from those downs faster. Further, when you have conflicting thoughts and beliefs, it acts as a mediator that eliminates the conflict. Whatever thought and belief clashes don't align with the goal(s) are laid to rest, and those that enforce it gain more importance in your mind.

GOD-GIVEN MEDICINE (HEALING FROM THE UNIVERSAL INTELLIGENCE)

In this section, I will discuss my personal opinion when it comes to healing. You might have different beliefs, but I hope I can provide new perspectives that can contribute to yours. I believe God made it possible for us to live healthily and happily with a high quality of life using natural means. I believe this applies to all of your health, from above-down, inside-out. Our health, happiness, and quality of life are determined by what we put in, on, and around our bodies physically, chemically, and emotionally. It's simple, but it requires that you have the necessary knowledge about the health resources you have available. Some of these means are resources down in this section.

Water is an essential tool for healing. It's required for us to live, and it's needed for many other species to live, from microbes to blue whales. When you don't drink enough water, your body weakens, and you don't last as long in the physical tasks that you're trying to accomplish. But, when you routinely drink enough water, your body can clean itself and provide the liquids needed to carry out internal chemical reactions. With the chemical reactions functioning as they're supposed to, your body will have better overall health, and it will have much more energy to carry out the tasks you're trying to do.

Eating whole foods gives you the energy you need to get work done. It also provides the minerals, vitamins, and other nutrients necessary for the body to carry out the processes it needs to live healthily. If you don't eat healthily (such as eating processed foods routinely, not eating enough, having too much sugar, etc.), you're opening yourself up to a range of various health concerns. Similarly, herbs and plants can provide healing chemicals that are necessary to recover from a large variety of medical conditions. These range from life-changing conditions to minor daily nuisances like a runny nose.

You need to spend time outside in nature. You need sunlight for good health. Without it, you would be hard-pressed to properly process all the vitamins and nutrients your body needs. When you're unexposed to proper sunlight for extended periods, you'll become sickly and depressed. Grounding yourself is also highly beneficial to your health, particularly on a mental level. We need exposure to the natural world in order to keep our stress levels under control, mental health in check, and physical health under control. The same applies to having clean air to breathe. Clean air isn't just necessary for your body's chemical processes but also exerts a strong beneficial effect on your mental health (particularly in relation to anxiety levels).

Your body needs movement and exercise to maintain its muscle tone and for the body to function well overall. The movement can't just be something you do now and then. It needs to happen on a daily basis. Exercise, taking walks, moving about, and stretching are all critical for your body to function at an optimal level. And if you want your body and mind to operate at tip-top performance, it requires dedicated daily exercise, action, and mobility work. This is even better if you can get the body in motion outside in the elements and surrounded by nature.

Conscious breathwork is necessary for anyone trying to deal with the anxieties and stresses of life. Normal breathing brings oxygen into your body, without which you wouldn't be alive for more than a few minutes. It's also essential as a way to get rid of carbon dioxide so that it doesn't pile up in the body as a waste product. With smooth flows of clean air coming in and used air going out, your body can carry out the chemical reactions it needs to function effectively. Conscious breathing helps to slow down your heartbeat and respiratory rate to find yourself in a more parasympathetic state. This is best done by taking time to be present with your breath. Breathe in through your nose and let your stomach expand outwardly. Breathe out through your nose as you feel your stomach fall. Visualize the air coming into your body as your lungs expand and leaving your body as the lungs deflate. This can be done whenever you need to help regulate your nervous system.

Meditation, gratitude, and keeping a positive perspective are essential forms of medicine for your mind that translate into health benefits for your body. With meditation, you coach your body to work at a homeostatic level, and you bring your mind into a calmer state. Gratitude gets you to the point where you recognize all the good in your life, and you acknowledge the positive effects that have been had because of it. Holding a positive perspective keeps you focused on what's really important—the good that you and others can (and do) contribute to the world.

Cold exposure, specifically cold showers or ice baths, is something that you can utilize on a daily basis to help improve mood, increase energy and have fewer feelings of inflammation in your body. I feel more motivated, disciplined, and energized than ever before because I make the consistent and conscious choice every day to get out of my comfort zone and do cold exposure. Cold exposure has also been shown to enhance overall health and longevity, improve sleep quality and reduce pain. I suggest taking it slow when you start because it will shock your nervous system. A good breathwork routine is essential before you start cold exposure, but once you have that, you can begin experiencing the many benefits.

Lack of sleep is one of the fastest-acting health depreciators. When you don't have enough sleep, you can almost instantly start to see the results in how you behave and how your body feels. On the flip side, you function well when you routinely get enough quality rest. You are alert mentally—sleeping well by routinely getting enough hours, having a consistent sleeping time, and not being exposed to electronics right before bed.

Reading is medicine for the mind. You cannot become a new person without a new mindset and a new perspective. One of the quickest ways to gain a new perspective in our current reality is through mediums such as books and audiobooks. You learn and therefore become more adept as an individual. You also gain new perspectives that help you see the world from more than just one point of view. Problem-solving improves because you learn ways that others solve problems, ways that you might not have thought of or used. Then there are the health benefits of lower stress, lightening depression, and improving your quality of sleep (Stanborough, 2019).

The power that made the body heals the body. When you have faith in a higher power or Universal Intelligence, you can rely on that in your healing process rather than the fear that you won't get better or that you will die if you don't follow through with healing practices. This changes your perspective from a fear-based one to a faith-based one. Further, when you have faith and morals that align with that faith, you can't go around telling people to behave in a certain way when you don't behave in that way—practice what you preach.

We need to have our human values of honesty, kindness, generosity, work ethic, and tolerance at the forefront of our minds on a daily basis. When we do, we make the world a healthier place for ourselves and others. By exerting some self-control and having integrity, we set an example of good behavior that makes our social interactions easier and healthier. We are a social species, and with social relations being so crucial to mental health, there's an excellent reason to keep our values at the forefront of our minds on a daily basis. By doing so, our subconscious will be induced into behavior that's appropriate to those values.

ACTION STEP

Speak in the present tense, particularly when you're saying your affirmations. They're not something that's going to happen in the future but rather something that you're bringing into existence right now. And realize that it's not far-fetched that you're busy making your goals a reality. You are worthy of achieving your worthwhile dreams—any hidden thoughts that you don't deserve happiness, success, and achievement no longer deserve your attention. So, affirm your goals in the present every day and focus on the thoughts, sensations, and perceptions you have as you have those goals achieved. This action step will gradually align your subconscious mind to the things you want to bring into reality.

3

THE EGO

> *"The moment you become aware of the ego in you, it is strictly speaking no longer the ego, but just an old, conditioned mind pattern. Ego implies unawareness. Awareness and ego cannot coexist."*
>
> — ECKHART TOLLE

IS EGO REALLY THE ENEMY?

The ego gets a bad rap. Many people call the ego the enemy but being able to learn about and understand the ego is how we can learn to improve our overall health and well-being. The ego doesn't live in the present. It's a part of the mind that operates in the past and uses past data to defend you. It also uses the future so that you can escape your present reality and imagine the great things you're going to be and do. The present isn't the realm of the ego. It's the realm where you have control. By understanding your ego, understanding your past and its influence on you, and grasping the future, you can create using your present reality. You'll be in much better shape as an individual.

To distill the basics of the ego, it is the "I" of the mind. It is you and the way you see yourself as an identity between your base desires and your ethical identity. Your personality, along with the beliefs you hold, the habits that identify you, and the traits you represent, are identifiable with your ego. It's an unconscious part of the mind that tries to act as you do, but with the purpose of defending you and your interests from dangers, risks, or unwanted situations.

The ego uses your perceptions of the external world to record the experience for you to remember at a later stage. The perceptions you have at present and the input you receive are evaluated by the ego so that it can plan its courses of action based on past events. The courses of action it dictates impact both the physical world around you and your social environment. Your ego can dictate what you should do in a social situation if it perceives that you should react in a certain pre-programmed way for your own benefit and safety.

So, let's say you're in a social situation where there's an angry security guard that's upset about the way you've parked. In the past, you've seen someone throw a tantrum when confronted by an official, leading to the official's manager resolving the situation. Thus, your ego uses that same course of action to determine that you should be rude, angry, and upset. Like a wound-up doll, you do exactly what your ego has instructed, and the confrontation ends. Thus, the ego is validated in using that past-term observed action and will use it as a defense mechanism in similar situations in the future.

The other two agencies of the mind are the id and superego. The id is the part of the mind that contains all your desires. The urges you have (whether acted on or not) are contained in it. The superego contains all the moral regulations and the code of conduct you should use as an individual. It regulates the urges of the id so that you don't act on those urges that would be considered immoral.

The ego serves as a buffer between the two and decides the course of action to be taken. It's the "leader" of the mind that determines what will be done in a given situation. It considers the ethical arguments of the superego when making its decisions. It also considers the desires the id would like to carry out. Let's look at this playing out in an example.

You've just come face to face with the person you know who has shamelessly been flirting with your spouse at their job.

Your id presents its desire to rip them a new one and assault them for everyone on the premises to see. Your superego presents moral and ethical considerations such as not being violent, not damaging someone's reputation without established evidence, etc. Ultimately, your ego considers both points and decides on a balance between the two—you raise your voice at the person out of earshot from other people in the company, and you make a fuss, but you don't assault them. The ego acted as the leader here and used historical experiences to conclude it wouldn't be advisable to break the law but that it is satisfying to speak your mind when you've been wronged.

The ego can be seen as a relay point between the inner and outer worlds. By taking in the stimuli of the world around you, it can control your various functions (like your motor activity, your thinking, planning, judgment, and so forth) to implement actions of the past in your best interests. It's an expert at using the stimulus-response mechanism, using this tool to see what actions produced the highest personal rewards and what actions produced the highest amount of pain or punishment. As a result, it's an effective tool to handle unwanted stimuli for you in ways that would be acceptable to your sensibilities. It refines its courses of action over the years using this crude sense of learning and logic.

The reason the ego gets a bad name is when its sense of identity isn't very strong, when it acts impulsively, and when it responds with a distorted sense of reality. This is because of an inferiority complex in many cases. The person in question isn't confident in their capabilities or identity, and they're faced with situations they don't want to face or handle. The ego jumps in to take over and protect them, resulting in it having authority in the situation. The person isn't really involved in the problem and the actions taken, and they're not providing their input into the situation since the ego is doing it for them. As such, there might be some distortions from their personality in terms of how to react when presented with similar problems (i.e., seemingly impulsive behavior).

This weak ego is more and more involved with its own schemes, interpretations, and activities as it takes over things for the person. It doesn't have accurate concepts of the self (you) because it's not in direct contact with you in all situations, seeing that you've withdrawn from handling some types of problems yourself. As a result, it starts seeing itself in all sorts of ways that you might not see yourself, ranging from neurotic to grandiose. Because it's so occupied with maintaining this identity for you (the identity it's constructed), it becomes lazy or unproductive on other matters that seem less important to it.

On the other hand, there's the case of a strong ego that's an asset to your inner world. It's not overly influenced by the id when it comes to desires and does not act impulsively in an attempt to protect your identity and your survival. It takes in information and objectively compares it to past experiences to formulate well-thought-out plans. Those plans are developed and implemented as distinct from the environmental pressures (including social pressures) you're facing, making it possible for the ego's solutions to be long-term oriented rather than used for short-term benefit. As its solutions are well-thought-out, there isn't much reason to veer off from what they suggest—its recommendations are reliable and decisive.

DISADVANTAGES OF THE EGO

The main advantages of the ego are a result of the ego being in a weak state of having an altered sense of identity. The distorted self-reality results in confusion on your part when you notice yourself doing things that you don't want to do. Or, on some occasions, you might do things you would disagree with, but you don't even notice or remember them because the ego came to "save the day" by standing in your place in a situation that would have given you discomfort. You hear about this sort of thing in cases where someone went into a fit of rage and did something ridiculous, followed by having the experience as a blank in their mind. The ego "protected" them (by attacking the threat) so that they could remove themselves from having to face the situation.

Another problem with the ego is that it's stuck in its ways. The solutions it uses are affirmed to it as reasonable solutions when they produce a result that it finds acceptable. It then keeps on using that type of solution in future situations with similar stimuli. In a world that's changing fast in terms of material advances, mental health technology, social contexts, human rights, and prioritization of the Earth's sustained existence, being stuck in your ways is a problem. When you want to get out of your comfort zone and change things up, the ego pushes back and reaffirms the necessity to use its tried and tested solutions. The result is cognitive dissonance–you can't decide whether it would be better to change or stay the same.

You can counteract the ego's resistance to change. To do this, you need to do some introspection so that you understand the reasons you're not changing. Find the memories, beliefs, thoughts, habits, and fears that dictate you should stay as you are. Break them apart by observing them because the confrontation between you and your conscious mind can lead you to cancel out the need for those things to continue existing. When you've seen why they are in place, you can replace them with the beliefs, ideas, habits, etc., that you wish to bring in as a change, with the goal or purpose behind the change being the fuel for the ego to change. Your mind will bend to your will if you observe its shortcomings directly, you affirm the changes you want to instill, and you keep your motivation for change at the forefront of your mind.

There are perceived benefits for the ego to stay the same in addition to the use of already proven successes with those courses of action. One of these is that you will be perceived as normal when you stick to what's known. If you change, it could seem odd to others, resulting in you becoming ostracized. Further, if you change the way you do things, you might violate the expectations others have of you. It might be in your best interests to go against those expectations, but if you do, you might feel guilty (which is something the ego would prefer you don't go through).

Then there's the matter of success and failure. When you do something new, you might cause yourself to fail along a certain line. The "winning formula" is violated, which is something the ego doesn't want to do, as this could expose you to potential risk. Likewise, the change could bring about unprecedented success. If it does, then you might have to face conditions and people you're not mentally, emotionally, and educationally prepared for. Many people fear too much success as much as failure (even if they won't admit it directly). As Marianne Williamson once said, "Our deepest fear is not that we are inadequate. Our deepest fear is that we are powerful beyond measure."

THE FIVE STEPS OF EGO-WORK

In this section, we're going to look at the steps you can take to improve the synergy between you and your ego.

The first step is to have an introduction to the ego. This is made possible by getting yourself in a comfortable place and position, then affirming that you're going to observe the ego. Affirm to yourself that you will see it as separate from yourself. This is because, up to this point, you've likely been associating its behavior with yourself and vice versa when you're two separate entities. The next step is to become more observant of the way you communicate (both to yourself and others). The way you communicate after using the word "I" is ego-speak. The words you say, how you say them, and the communication being given between the lines. Observing these things over a period of a few days is an easy way to get to know your ego in a more humble way.

Once you've had some good encounters with your ego, you should name it. This emphasizes the separateness between you and it. An essential aspect of working on your ego is that you're able to examine it objectively. When the separateness of it is emphasized, it's easier to look at it in an unbiased way.

The fourth step is to observe how your ego operates when it's triggered. This step should only be done when the action of getting to know your ego (by listening to the "I" statements) has been done for a few weeks. To do this step, note when you're in a situation where your emotions are excessively strong or negative. See what the stimulus was for the excessive reaction (such as your child leaving their sports equipment lying on the floor after their shower). When you see what the trigger was, determine why you reacted in the way you did. In this case, leaving the equipment on the floor makes you feel like your child thinks you're there to clean up after them and that your time is less important than theirs. Once you've determined what the underlying feeling was, it should ease because you see that either the reaction was unnecessary or that you need to have a conversation with the other person so that they know how the action makes you feel. The ego overreacts like this sometimes because it doesn't know how to handle the situation, so instead of trying to deal with the difficult or frustrating situation, it takes out the emotions that are triggered in someone. In many cases, the person who receives the brunt of the emotions isn't even involved with the situation but just a convenient outlet (such as a boss shouting at their employees when they've just had an argument with their wife).

The final step is to change the way you react to triggering situations. This is done by feeling gratitude to your ego for trying to protect you from the underlying feeling caused by the situation (the sense that the parent's time isn't valuable in the example with the sports equipment). Figure out how you would like to react to situations like that in the future, then tell yourself that it would be acceptable to respond in the newly selected way when faced with similar problems in the future (this acts as a positive command that the ego should comply with). The parent could say that it would be okay for them to react with indifference when confronted with sports equipment lying around in the future. They should then state to themselves that it's unnecessary to attach the underlying feeling to the same situation in the future because there isn't a connection between the problem, what they're feeling and what was done. The child most likely had other things on their mind and forgot about equipment; they didn't think their time was more important than their parent's.

There is an extra step you can take to cleanse your ego of triggers and unwanted reactions. Attend a lecture about a topic you don't like or a gathering of a group you don't like. Alternatively, watch videos or listen to radio transmissions from people you disagree with. Listen and note when you feel triggered. Note what concepts triggered you and what the underlying feelings were that developed from those triggers. Note them down, so you can go back afterward to work through them. Please go through the list and do the fourth and final steps with each one of them. Work through all the triggers and replace the underlying ideas and feelings with ones that would be more appropriate to similar conversations and situations. In doing so, you're bringing your reactions back under control and asserting your dominance when it comes to situations that make you uncomfortable.

The ego has an identity that has little to no fluidity. It's defensive and is stuck in the beliefs and patterns that it created. It fights against things that go against those patterns or ideas and becomes defensive in order to protect you. The steps above are how you can identify those stuck points that are inappropriate to a situation and how to replace them with more appropriate emotions and reactions to use in the future.

You are the control point of your mind, body, and life. Your ego needs to accept what you tell it to do, but likewise, you need to accept it for being what it is and operating as it does. Only by seeing it fully will you be able to change it.

ACTION STEP

A simple step you can take right now to start softening your ego and making the process of re-exerting control of your life is simply to ask yourself who you are. Who are you when no one is watching, and does it align with who you want to be? Work out all the things that form part of your identity (as you see yourself, not as others tell you to see yourself or how they say they see you). You don't have to make a list but should instead look at the traits you have and examine yourself with a curious mindset. Don't make it too serious; keep yourself in a state of light curiosity and review yourself. By bringing yourself more in touch with yourself, you'll see what behavior and statements from you are not really you but part of your ego or the other parts of your subconscious mind. You can do this exercise for a few minutes every day until you feel calmly acquainted with yourself and more comfortable with your identity.

4

STOICISM

"You could leave life right now. Let that determine what you do and say and think."

— MARCUS AURELIUS

WHAT ARE YOU AFRAID OF?

The philosophy of Stoicism was first introduced to me in early 2018 after my father had a massive heart attack. It was the paradigm-shifting moment in my life. We hear stories every day about someone else's loved one having a severe health incident, but it's never your loved one. Until one day, it is. Luckily, my dad lived through the experience after being intubated for six days and having the ER doctor visit him on day 7 to tell him that he wanted to see him for himself because he didn't think he was going to make it. This experience pushed me to seek a mental health counselor for the first time in my life. After months of therapy, I realized that my dad's heart attack, the worst thing that had ever happened to me at that point in my life, was arguably the best thing to have ever happened to me. It allowed me to look in the mirror and ask if I was okay and if my current actions aligned with my desired values and beliefs. It allowed me to seek help. It allowed me to work through past traumas, childhood conditioning, and insecurities by going and talking to someone. Most importantly, it allowed me to heal and be at peace with our mortality.

A BRIEF HISTORY OF STOICISM

Stoicism is a philosophy that was initially founded in Greece more than 2,300 years ago. It was founded at a time when Greece and its city-states were no longer the most powerful forces in the world. Individual liberty had been replaced by the Roman idea of the group being all and the individual living to serve the group. It was influenced by the philosophies and teachings that came before it, but with many changes and advances. This was for those who subscribed to it to see the world in a way that was appropriate to modern times. The philosophies of old were no longer completely relevant to the world where Stoicism was born.

The beliefs of the Stoics were originally centered around there being value in living a life of simplicity, not getting emotionally caught up in things, and the importance of looking at the world logically. The founder of this philosophy was Zeno of Citium, a philosophy student who had studied at Plato's Academy and who had written much on the subject of philosophy before founding Stoicism. He was known for emphasizing ethics, logic, and physics as the three main divisions of the subject of philosophy. This allowed students to see philosophy in a more structured way and allowed them to build on their current understanding of the field.

One of the core beliefs underlying this original rendition of Stoicism was the importance of logic as an instrument in handling the affairs of our life. The proper course of action would be worked out using reasoning. A person who was wise was considered to be the aspiration all should strive for, as wisdom meant that a person could overcome the challenges they faced, and they would do so using the knowledge they had formed a certainty on. Wisdom included living in accordance with the natural order, and if you lived in such a way, you would bring about a life of happiness.

Chrysippus, one of the earliest Stoics, expanded a lot on philosophy. He stated that reasoning wasn't just essential for living happily but also for discerning between good and evil. Goodness was when you acted in alignment with both human nature and the nature of the world (i.e., he broke down the natural order into two distinct parts that people could think logically with). He pointed out how it's essential to use self-preservation as a criterion in your thinking and actions—survival is a core part of both human nature and the nature of the world.

The Romans took on Stoicism, which became popular with them, mainly because they had a very practical outlook on life and doing things. During this time, Stoicism centered more on religion and morals. In terms of morals, there was a focus on the importance of duty, the law, and divine reasoning. It was believed that there were basic rules underlying the way the world operated and that it was obliged to live in accordance with them. By the time Christianity had become popular in Ancient Rome, much of the Stoic way of thinking, reasoning, arguing, and looking at life had become widespread practice amongst all classes of Rome.

As Christianity became the central religion in Rome, Stoicism was heavily criticized by some early Christian opinion leaders. Despite this, there were many outlooks of the Church that the Stoics influenced, and there were many points of the Christian belief system that were in line with Stoicism. One of these was that humans all share a bond and originate from the same universal source—they carried the energy of the divine. In line with this, both linked the human soul to the supernatural, with the soul being viewed as being extended from the divine. The divine (in other words, God) was considered to be natural and governed the way the natural world exists. Another core belief of both ideologies at the time was that truth is obtainable by basing it on other truths (i.e., lies don't lead to the truth).

As the Middle Ages arrived, there were more clashes between Stoicism and Christianity. One such clash was when the Stoics questioned how God could be angry and express wrath when God wasn't enslaved to the passions. However, Stoicism started being applied to other areas and was no longer used as a major comparison tool for Christian beliefs. It had become an important philosophy for analyzing political philosophy, social philosophy, and the different types of laws, in addition to its earlier use for analyzing religion and logic. An earlier belief of the philosophy that came to the forefront once more was the difference between civil, natural, and national law. During this age, Stoicism was thus expanded into multiple fields that were new or that were being revitalized in relation to living in accordance with the natural order.

Stoicism has remained relevant since the Renaissance. Some of its basic principles are important in other philosophies and in everyday thinking. These principles include determination of your own actions, using reasoning to solve problems in a logical way, that acting with virtue is good while falling prey to temptation is evil, and that we need to exert self-control so that we remain in command of our emotions.

MEMENTO MORI

"Memento mori" is a stoic saying that means "remember you must die" and serves as a reminder that death will happen, no matter what. The purpose of this reminder is to remember to value life because death might take it away at any time. When we know things might end and that it's not a given that we're going to live a long life, we realize that the time we have every day should hold importance for us. And the time we do have available will be spent much better when we've faced and overcome our deepest fears.

Napoleon Hill described six basic fears in his book *Outwitting the Devil*. Overcoming these fears will give you much more strength and happiness. Your quality of living will be higher because you won't concern yourself with fears but rather with life. The six fears Napoleon Hill listed were the fear of loss of love, fear of old age, fear of poverty, fear of criticism, fear of ill health, and fear of death. You'll feel immense relief with any one of these fears overcome, but here we're going to focus on the fear of death.

When we know that we're mortal, we know that we shouldn't take our time for granted. Wasting the time we have doesn't help anyone, particularly ourselves. Reflecting on our impending death might be morbid and depressing, but it's a fact of life. The sooner we confront it and accept that it's going to happen, the sooner we can bring our attention to the fact that we should live using the time that we have. If we reflect on this daily for a minute or so, we instill the motivation we need to make the most out of the day.

I wear a pendant around my neck every day that says "Memento Mori." It's close to my heart and serves as a reminder that this life is temporary. It motivates me to live a healthy lifestyle and to do what I can to create happiness. If I can stop living at any moment, then I need to dedicate the gift of time that I have available to pursue my goals and happiness for myself and others. Sometimes we need a reason to get up and take action rather than sitting back and being lazy—memento mori serves this purpose. I owe it to my wife and children to be the absolute best version of myself with the time that I have here on Earth.

I have come to terms with the fact that I might die at some moment near the present or far in the future. Knowing that it's part of life and that life is brief helps me to realize that I'm being given the same opportunity as everyone else. Life is fragile and precious, and it's that way for everyone. So, be grateful for what you have. Even if it isn't all you want, you have time, and you have the people and things around you in the present. Honor those that have come before you by using the time you've been given to be the best version of yourself.

DEATH AND MORTALITY

It seems counterintuitive, but thinking about death and mortality can improve our quality of life. The experience might not be pleasant because we're facing the fact that we might lose everyone and everything we love, and there's nothing we can do about it. Despite the experience being depressing, it can be uplifting. It's uplifting because we realize that everyone will go through the same thing and that we're not at that point yet. We have a lot to be thankful for, and we have a lot that we can still do while we're here. The "scarceness" of the time we have left makes it that much more worthwhile.

When you know that you and your loved ones don't have a limitless amount of time left, you realize that there's no point in wasting the time you have or taking the time you have with loved ones for granted. You're going to take hold of the time you have left and use it to pursue the things you find important. Thus, your life will be lived more authentically, and you will live more in line with your beliefs and values. As a result, your life will be lived more positively because you know you're being true to yourself. Thinking about death and mortality for a few minutes each day might not be pleasant, but it's worth it in the long run.

HOW DO YOU WANT TO BE REMEMBERED?

Of course, when you know that you're going to die at one point or another, the question arises about what you want your legacy to be. Do you want to be remembered for certain achievements, for the values and personality you embodied in your daily living, for the people who are close to you, or something else? Asking yourself how you want to be remembered puts it all in perspective. It puts the things that you consider the most important at the forefront of your consideration. The question puts a lot of motivation in your mind from the start of the day to the end because you know that everything you're doing is going to contribute to your legacy.

Having this in our minds every day will change us from being complacent to being action-driven. When we know that we have power over the things and memories we leave behind, then we can act intentionally to make those things and memories good. You gain a lot of clarity when you ask yourself the question, "how do I want to be remembered when I die?" It clarifies what you think is important and helps you define your identity.

Having your desired end result in perspective is a good way of bringing you into the present. There are things that you want in the future, but you know that you'll only get them by focusing on what you're doing right now to advance toward that future. With reduced confusion about your identity, long-term desires, and values, you can jump into any task with a level of certainty in your mind.

TRAUMA AND LIFE STRUGGLE

Trauma is that overwhelming sense of emotion that we feel when we've gone through a horrible life experience. This can happen in all sorts of situations, such as when a family member passes on, when sexual abuse takes place, or when you go and lose everything you've worked for in your life. When you go through such an experience, it's common for you to sit with the event unprocessed for quite a while. In many cases, it takes people years to work through a traumatic experience to the point where they can comfortably face the memory of it.

Some of the things you can expect to experience before you've worked through trauma are shock, emotionlessness, overwhelming surges of emotion, flashbacks in which you relive the trauma, deteriorating relationships (particularly with those somehow connected to the event), and unpleasant body sensations or conditions. Many who have gone through real trauma might bottle up the experience entirely and pretend that it didn't occur. But don't you ask them about the experience because you're bound to get back a cold response of it not being your business or that the person is "fine."

We can't go through our lives living with these feelings and reactions. Everyone goes through trauma during their lives —and in many cases, at multiple points in their lives. As harsh as it might sound, we can choose to either sink or swim. We can let the waves overwhelm us and let us go under, or we can use coping techniques to face up to the situation to our and others' benefit. If we choose to swim, we become much stronger as individuals. It's not clear when a traumatic event first happens and when we're still working through it, but the situation happened for us, not to us. We become stronger, more appreciative of the life we have, and grow in many facets of our lives. This is called post-traumatic growth.

We need to learn that our choices are always going to affect us, even those choices we make when we're down and angry at the world. How we choose to respond to the situation will determine whether we rise to greater heights and do justice after the trauma or whether we will let the trauma take advantage of us and bring us down. Remember that the traumatic experience isn't going to fix itself. You're going to have to take what you can out of the incident and use it to your advantage, no matter how messed up the situation was. We can motivate others to become better people who aim higher and work to achieve their dreams. There's something about a person who's gone through hell but has risen above it to achieve at higher levels that will always inspire others.

And if you can't face the situation at first and stumble along your path of overcoming the trauma, that's okay. You don't have to rise up out of it like a phoenix from the ashes. You're an individual with the right to live your own experiences and work through them on your own terms. Those times you fall down along your recovery should serve as lessons you learn from. If you fell in with the wrong crowd because you hated the world and find yourself in a dark place you don't want to be a few weeks, months, or years later, then learn from that. Choose a new crowd of people that will uplift you and negate the presence of the wrong crowd in your life. Your lesson was to not fall in with that group of people, so use it and rise up. If you stumble again, then gently pick up the pieces and keep working on advancing. You're a human with immense capacity for changing your situations in life.

Over time, failing and picking yourself up will make you stronger and stronger. If you rose up from the experience like a phoenix with no stumbles along the way, then you've made yourself stronger that much faster. The critical thing to remember is that there are many emotions related to trauma, and how we choose to face them or not face them can make us weaker or stronger.

AFTER ACCEPTING YOUR FEARS

Accepting your fears is the difficult first step suggested in this chapter. This starts by recognizing what your fears are and their extent. Please don't run away from them; instead, observe what makes you feel scared or anxious and note it down. There may be many things on your list, and that's okay. Most people have multiple sources of fear. When you've got them all (or you think you've got them all), accept that you have fears and tell yourself that it's okay to have them. You can study different ways to accept your fears and techniques to reduce your fears. But here, we're going to leave it at a level of acceptance and then look at how to grow above those fears.

The way to rise above your fears is to look at the opposite of each fear and then put your focus on that. So, if you fear failing a college class and losing a scholarship, instead focus on doing well and learning from the textbooks and lectures you're studying. Remember that the subconscious mind plays an essential role in how we act and the results we bring about in life. It follows the direction we tell it to, so when we focus on the opposite of our fears, then it will do what it can to make the opposite become a reality.

So, as a first step, focus on abundance. There's an abundance of money, things, friends, love, and connection in your life. While we might not feel we have a lot, we often have much more than we think. People often look at our lives with envy, while we don't realize how much more we have than them. And even if we don't have a lot, we can use creative visualization to motivate ourselves as to what our lives would be like with more. For example, if we don't yet have a lot of friends because we're new to an area, we can meditate on the hypothetical experience of a bunch of our friends that we're going to make in the next few months visiting at our home and enjoying their time with us. Then we have a destination to work towards; we're focusing on what we want to occur rather than the fact that we don't have that just yet.

Appreciation is another thing to focus on. There's a whole chapter in this book dedicated to gratitude and its power in our lives—for good reason. Appreciate the skills you have, the values you hold, and your identity as a whole. When you do, you're reinforcing them and empowering yourself. When you focus on your shortcomings, you'll likely end up depressing yourself and losing sight of all your capabilities. If you do the converse, you'll raise your confidence and get much more done.

Love is something that creates a lot of goodness in our lives —the love of the people close to our families and us. We can extend it further to our love for the things we do and the various living things in our lives (such as our pets and plants). When someone doesn't like what they do, they can change that by envisioning the things they do love about what they do. For instance, if you're a lab assistant and hate your job, change your perspective and see what you love about it. Perhaps you have a good schedule that allows you to have a reasonable work-life balance. Spot all the good things about what you do and be grateful for them. I also love using the example of going to someone's social media that you don't like. Take time to look at their life and think about things that you love, admire, appreciate or respect about their existence. This can be a challenging but beneficial experience for you to heal from built-up angst toward another human that is more than likely just trying to figure out the world like you are. Soon you'll find that things become less unbearable, and you will actually enjoy your life and its activities more.

A healthy person has a thousand wishes. An unhealthy person has only one. Being healthy is something that makes your life much easier. When you're unhealthy or ill, it can put a lot of strain on you and those close to you. If you have a condition, see what you can do about it, and run with that. You're going to overwhelm yourself with hopelessness if you focus on the bad and the things you can't fix. I've seen this with many of my patients that have had cancer—while they knew they were on a path that would likely lead to death, they kept on looking at what they could still do and being grateful for the health they had left. If they could still walk, they would be grateful and use that capability to keep their body exercised and stay motivated about seeing people they like. If they could no longer walk, they would focus on the fact that they weren't bedridden but could get around using a wheelchair. This capacity to see the good in their health always serves as an inspiration. It is something that inspires me every day. I will always remember them, and I never take my health for granted because of it.

Focus on the long-term rather than the short-term. There might be a few setbacks now and then. That doesn't mean they're permanent. Our actions and their results affect our lives and our legacy. Keep looking at the results you're creating in the long run because you do have the capacity to cause long-term results. Focus on longevity because if we do, we'll make choices that are right for our health, happiness, and quality of life over the long run. Keep your whole life view at the forefront, always.

The most significant focus should be on life. While we look at death and mortality, we do this to appreciate the life that we have. Our life is a gift that we can use as we see fit. We can use it for selfish, harmful, or destructive reasons, or we can use it for constructive and positive purposes. If we look at physics, then matter, energy, space, and time make up the universe. It is said that energy cannot be destroyed, and it is also said that we are made up of energy on a spiritual level. In other words, it can be declared that death is an illusion and that there is eternal life in this universe. Whether this is true or not isn't something that can be determined with certainty right now. But, it is reassuring to think that we're part of the endlessness of the universe and will remain a part of it on some level long after our bodies have perished.

Focusing on the positive things noted in this section makes you far happier and more driven in life. Your fears are valid, but you don't have to focus on them.

ACTION STEP

Take a moment to reflect on your life. There are many things you have gone through, some of them unpleasant or traumatic. Isolate one of those incidents and reflect on what happened in it. Please don't go too deep because the purpose isn't to relive it. After seeing what happened in the incident, take a broader look and see how it affected you later in life. Look at the emotional, financial, physical, and spiritual effects that the event had on you. Look at the positive—the silver lining, if you will. See how you changed and how you became stronger. Look at how you've changed your thinking so that you avoid getting into the same situation again. Go through all the positive effects you can see and acknowledge that, in many ways, the experience had a positive impact on you. This might be a painful exercise, but it's gratifying.

5

CREATIVE VISUALIZATION

"We always attract into our lives whatever we think about most, believe most strongly, expect on the deepest level, and imagine most vividly."

— SHAKTI GAWAIN

CAN YOU SEE IT HEALED?

The first step to healing is believing that you can be healed. Creative visualization is the practice of seeing something in your mind's eye. The purpose is to have an emotional effect or to provide you with motivation. The practice of creative visualization is often done in line with meditation and breathing exercises. One of the unexpected benefits of visualization is that you can create a healing environment for your body and your mind.

One of the tricks with a proper creative visualization technique is that you need to visualize the things you're seeing as if they're happening right now. It needs to be in real-time in your mind's eye. In other words, you're going to go through all the perceptions you would feel as if you're feeling them right now. You're going to imagine the people, places, and yourself as you would look at the time in the future when the creative visualization event ought to take place. I tapped into this years ago before realizing what I was doing. Before I met my wife, I lived in downtown Indianapolis, and I would take walks by myself, listening to calming, chill music in my headphones. As I walked, I would visualize her next to me, holding my hand. I would think about how happy she made me and how grateful I was to have found her in my life. I would feel all of those feelings in the present moment. I knew that she existed already. It gave me peace and allowed me to focus on becoming the best version of myself while I waited for her to come into my life. By holding the creative visualization in the present moment, you're working on creating it into a reality.

When you visualize, you need to be exact because you're putting an instruction out to the universe of what you want to come true. You're manifesting what you want and doing it in such a way that full details are given. And don't be shy about being as positive as you want to be. If you can't face it in your own mental world (the full image of success), then how will you bring the full state of success into reality?

When you've done a session in which you visualize what you want, it's helpful to re-visualize it on a daily basis. In that way, you keep on creating towards it and prioritizing that future reality as something you want to bring into existence. Not only will this send out the signals into the universe you want, but it will also keep it as a priority in both your conscious and subconscious minds. Suppose you want to be an executive in your company in ten years. In that case, you need to keep visualizing that reality daily to make appropriate decisions and take necessary actions to have that come into existence. In some ways, you can think of it as a goal with which you keep yourself motivated.

As a warning, don't put negativity into your creative visualization because you'll bring those negative things into reality alongside the positives. Or, if you place too much negativity into it, you won't achieve that visualization at all.

CREATIVE VISUALIZATION FOR PAIN RELIEF

Pain is a problematic condition that plagues many of us, whether young or old. Pain can be alleviated using the mind, and creative visualization is one of the best tools to accomplish this. If this concept is hard for you to believe or accept, that's fine. Keep reading.

To do this, you first need to make up your mind that you would like to be pain-free or that you would like to alleviate pain in a part of your body. When you do, then you have a purpose to work toward with the visualization technique. Find yourself a relaxing location and a good time of day to meditate and visualize. Waking up in the morning is as good a time as any, or going to bed. You know you won't be disturbed, and your body will be calm from the rest or in the process of calming down from the busy day. Doing it before you sleep should be much easier for you to rest after you've done meditative visualization. If you're trying to handle a severe or persistent issue, you should do multiple daily sessions (at least three for good and fast results).

At the start of your session, determine where the pain is and the level of the pain. Visualize it in your mind (with your eyes closed is easiest). Once you really feel it, erase that scene, then visualize the pain being replaced with a healthy, good condition. For this to happen, you can imagine any method—it doesn't have to be scientifically accurate. All you're doing is creating the image (with full perception) of transitioning from a painful condition into a healthy one. A visualization that isn't scientifically accurate but can be helpful is to see yourself pouring liquid fertilizer on a wound and watching the flesh and skin grow back.

Another helpful technique is dramatizing the condition, its parts, and the removal of the condition. You can imagine the pain, inflammation, or infection as a bunch of little characters. See their presence in your body and the effect they're creating. Then picture new characters coming in and defending the body by driving out the bad characters. This could be little white blood cells acting as soldiers and making bacteria leave through a cut. Another example is imagining little characters using a fire hose to blast cooling gel into an inflamed part of your body.

A third technique that you might find helpful is to use color visualization. Here, you would imagine your affected body part as the embodiment of a particular color (such as a bright red). Imagine the color and feel the sensations that go along with it. Then visualize a healing color, whatever it may be (a cool blue-green for purposes of an example). Feel the pain-free sensation and the vitality that forms from the healing color. Now see how the healing color gradually seeps into the body part and replaces the unhealthy, pain-ridden color.

Do these visualizations daily (or multiple times a day when serious) so that your mind gets the idea that you want that part of the body healed. At the end of each session, affirm to yourself that you see your visualization becoming a reality and confirm that you're healthier than you were. You'd be amazed at how well this creative visualization can speed recovery and reduce pain.

CREATIVE VISUALIZATION FOR STRESS AND ANXIETY

When you're doing creative visualization, on some level, you're using the law of attraction. What you're putting out, you're going to get back, and when you're putting out anxiety with your creative visualization, you will get back uncertain results. To prevent this from happening, you first need to reduce your stress and anxiety levels— in general and in relation to the goal you're trying to visualize creatively.

To start off with, you need to face reality as it is. If it's not an optimal situation, then observe it for what it is. Refrain from trying to evaluate the situation. Just look at it—unfounded negativity should be released. If it's a better situation than what you thought because you've been overthinking it, then look at it plainly. Now you have your current condition in hand, and you have a starting point to work from. If you have sources of negativity in your life and your environment (such as aggressive Twitter accounts or sensationalized news sites on your phone's notifications list), then cut them out. Unpleasant people who gossip, complain excessively, or criticize you for no reason should also be cut out to the degree you can. In essence, you're doing stress management. Protect your peace at all costs.

Once you've cut out stress sources and factually looked at things, you can do visualization techniques tailored to anxiety reduction. One of these is a brief visualization practice at the start of the day. Before you get out of bed:

1. Close your eyes and take a few deep breaths.
2. Picture all the things you have for the day and work through them in the order they're planned to happen.
3. When you see that you have uncertainty or stress regarding a planned event, see how you can alter the picture into a positive incident.
4. Be realistic about the positive image so that you can be confident that the day can occur in that way.

For instance, if you're nervous about giving a presentation at work, then picture how you can reasonably expect it to go (which might involve a few objections or criticisms), but picture how you handle each complaint confidently and to the satisfaction of the person who raised it. Do this with any planned event that gives rise to stress so that you feel calmer about your day and more ready to face it.

Another creative visualization method you can use at any time of day to reduce stress and anxiety is where you picture a peaceful scene. Set yourself up in a distraction-free environment and close your eyes. Picture a location that you imagine to be calm, such as a tranquil lake. Imagine yourself progressing along a route in the scene, like floating along the lake on a calm current. Notice the things around you. Imagine the rustling leaves of the bushes along the shore and the clouds drifting through the sky. This type of visualization brings you to your happy place and infuses you with calmness so that you can once more face the day. When you notice you've markedly calmed down, bring yourself back to the present, open your eyes, and breathe a few deep breaths.

When doing visualization for stress-reduction purposes, you're not necessarily going to cut out your stress all at once. But, you can reduce your levels of stress markedly. Thus, acknowledge the improvements that are made—being hard on yourself isn't going to reduce your anxiety any faster. Use breathwork throughout your visualization to keep your body oxygenated and ensure the parasympathetic system contributes to your relaxation. Be mindful of your visualizations and calmly make use of as many perceptions as you can.

ACTION STEP

Relax in a comfortable space that's as distraction-free as possible. You can lie down or sit, whichever you prefer. Please close your eyes so that it's easier to focus due to not taking in multiple visual cues. You're now going to do compassion visualization, wherein you can see yourself or another person with compassion and support.

If you want to use it on another person, select someone you've recently interacted with and felt ill will towards. Picture them in your mind and visualize them with as many qualities that they possess as you can. Now think of a mantra wherein you wish that person well, wish them kindness, and visualize them as embodying values you respect. Visualize yourself in a situation where that person represents the qualities that you approve of, and tell yourself that you enjoy this person's company. Do this for a while until you feel that you're calmly picturing the situation. Then, visualize the person as they usually behave and imagine yourself as having that same sense of calmness as you had in the previous visualization. Tell yourself that you tolerate the person as they are and that you exhibit good qualities, whether that person is acting amicably or otherwise.

To practice compassion visualization towards yourself:

1. Visualize yourself.
2. Picture the qualities you have and the mannerisms you use.
3. Tell yourself that you love yourself and that you respect who you are. If negative qualities come up, then tell yourself that you accept how you are and that you are a person who continually strives to be as good as you can be.

By repeating the above visualization practices daily or weekly, you'll find that you have less anxiety and feel greater love for yourself and others.

GRATITUDE

"Acknowledging the good that you already have in your life is the foundation for all abundance."

— ECKHART TOLLE

WHAT ARE YOU GRATEFUL FOR TODAY?

Gratitude is the feeling you feel when you're happy that something exists and you appreciate it. This is a very positive mindset because you're validating the good in your life rather than seeing the shortcomings. There's a lot of good, and when you feel gratitude for that good, then you're shifting your mind into a positive space. There are many benefits that can be had from doing this, including on a physical front.

Gratitude improves your level of happiness and heightens your general well-being (Harvard Health Publishing, 2021). Your relationships can be positively impacted by it, both romantic and social. It makes you and the other person relaxed enough to share things that would otherwise make you uncomfortable (such as criticisms, confusions, or disagreements.) This is mainly because expressing genuine gratitude to another increases the positive effect between both of you.

On a personal level, showing gratitude gives you a more thankful mindset. With this type of mindset, you have higher levels of motivation and feel more driven in your daily tasks. You realize there is good in the world that you and others can and do create. So by working diligently, you can generate more goodness for others to experience. This bonding between you and others is partly impacted by the release of oxytocin when you express gratitude (Mayo Clinic Health System, 2022).

Further, your mood is improved, resulting in fewer depressive feelings and lower levels of anxiety. When you have a positive mindset, your brain is signaled to think less negatively. It attempts to use new neural pathways that are more positive in nature, putting the older and more negative mindsets to rest (even if just for a while). This has physical effects, such as improving your quality of sleep, improving your immunity (thereby causing you to be less likely to pick up a disease), and it lightens the load of pain that you feel.

BEST WAYS TO PRACTICE IT DAILY

A visualization exercise is an excellent way to build on your gratitude because it gives you a high-quality experience of thankfulness. A simple visualization practice you can do is to think of all the things you're thankful for from the day. Re-experience the feeling from when you received the act, statement, help, etc., that you feel grateful for. Then, take a broader look and think about the things you're thankful for in general at the present moment. Acknowledge each thing that comes up and accept that you have it in your life.

Visualize the contributions you made to make that thing possible in your life. If you're thankful for your business operating at a successful level, visualize moments where you made material contributions to it, and thank yourself for those actions. Follow this by thinking of things external influences have contributed to your business, whether they be coworkers, employees, your spouse, nature, or God. Thank each of them when you visualize the contribution they made. Not only does this exercise improve your levels of gratitude, but it also strengthens your sense of certainty and stability regarding the business.

Thank others in your life, and do this genuinely. Don't restrict it to being thankful in your mind. And when you do thank people, don't only use words but put some meaning behind what you're saying. Use body language and appropriate voice inflection to show that you mean what you're saying. To really make the gratitude effective, try different ways of expressing it that might be relevant to the context. If you're in a staff meeting, expressing gratitude might be most effective by making an announcement regarding the person you're grateful towards so that everyone knows what they've done. In a family context, it might be most effective to leave a small handwritten note next to the person's bed with a small token of thanks (such as a chocolate to snack on or a caricature for them to laugh at).

A gratitude journal is a popular method of practicing gratitude. You write down the things you're grateful for, either on a daily or weekly basis. Times when good things happened or when people were helpful are the type of things to note down in your journal. You should note when someone tried to be helpful, even if they weren't entirely successful, because the fact that they were willing to be helpful shows that they were willing to give to you from themself. Visualizing the things you write down is helpful because you re-experience them, and you gain a boost of the emotion you felt in the moment. Some benefits of keeping a gratitude journal include improved sleep, lower levels of depression, and a more positive mindset.

You can work gratitude into your meditation and mindfulness practices as well. This is very easy to do with loving-kindness meditation. To use loving-kindness meditation in this way, think of a moment you had a good connection with someone and knew you felt a level of love or liking towards them. Isolate the feeling or emotion you felt at that moment. Let go of the moment, but hold onto the feeling. Bring those emotions into the present, holding them in suspension so that you really feel them. Label the feeling and direct it towards yourself until you feel good. Accept the emotion, forgive yourself for anything that needs forgiveness, feel gratitude towards yourself, and detach from the negativity you feel about yourself.

PRACTICING GRATITUDE FOR PAIN RELIEF

Gratitude reduces your pain levels, or at the very least, your perception of your pain levels. In addition to removing or reducing the sensation of pain, it contributes to your sense of well-being. This is particularly the case when you practice gratitude daily and if you do it for periods lasting between five minutes to half an hour.

Murphy and Rafie (2021) isolated a few gratitude exercises that are particularly effective at improving your sense of well-being by reducing your sensation of pain. These are described in this section.

A gratitude journal is the first exercise known to be really effective at this. Especially if you do the practice where you find three things each day that you're thankful for. You can extend this latter part to three things for the day, week, and year. Similar to your journal, you can write a gratitude letter to someone that you feel grateful to, whether they're in your life at present or no longer with you. It can be a relieving way to thank people that have passed on who you still have incomplete communication that you would like to converse with. If the person you're writing to is still in your life or alive, then consider sending it to them. If you have strained communication, that's okay—sending it might provide relief for you and them, even if it doesn't remedy the relationship. If you're on good terms, it will serve to strengthen your relationship.

Loving-kindness meditation, as described above, is very effective when it comes to lowering levels of pain. Positive word meditation is also known to produce this effect. To do positive word meditation, bring a word to mind that makes you feel good, strong, or positively oriented. Repeat the word to yourself at random points through the day when you're taking a break or you're feeling relaxed so that the word associates with those feelings. Later, you can use this word to slow your mind and body down and catch a breath by repeating it to yourself, which is perfect for starting off a meditation session in the right frame of mind. Follow this up by meditating in the present with your eyes closed and perceiving your body and environment. Repeat the word to yourself while meditating until you notice you're in a physically and emotionally calm state. You can open your eyes and end the meditation at this point.

PRACTICING GRATITUDE FOR STRESS AND ANXIETY

Gratitude brings down your anxiety levels and the tension you feel from stress by altering your thought patterns from negative ones to positive ones. It helps to establish and strengthen new neural pathways that replace old ones that weren't operating at a positive and capable level. You break down anxiety and stress by getting into the present because one of the defense mechanisms a mind uses against it is assumptions of the future or ruminating over events in the past. Thus, gratitude exercises that revolve around bringing you into the present with a thankful frame of mind are best at creating tranquility by overcoming anxiety.

The simplicity of this practice is to find something in the present you're thankful for. Look around you and see if there's anything in your presence that you're grateful for. Observe it mindfully by remaining aware of your body's sensations and your perceptions about the object, person, or condition in question. Focus on it or them and flow gratitude towards it in your mind's eye. Appreciate it and observe the beauty or goodness in it.

You can use grounding to really make sure that you're calm in the present. Feel the ground beneath your feet and observe the sights, sounds, smells, etc., around you. Once you've finished directing gratitude to the thing you've selected, appreciate the world you're in and expand that feeling so that you're cherishing the world that exists around you. Appreciate that you're alive and that there is a world you can live in and enjoy.

MY TAKE ON GRATITUDE

Gratitude is the best thing you can use to alter how you see the world. It makes you appreciate the beauty in the world around you. We all have so much to be grateful for. We all have something to appreciate, no matter how easy or difficult our lives are. But by spotting, acknowledging, and directing our gratitude towards it, we can generate higher levels of positivity and happiness in our lives. I start my day with gratitude to set the right tone for the rest of it. It begins with my alarm going off at 4:44 am, with my alarm labeled "take care of yourself" because I know I need to fill my cup first. Otherwise, I won't be able to pour myself into others' cups. The reason I chose 4:44 is because this is an angel number representing wholeness and love.

My morning routine is set up so that I know I've taken care of myself and that I have enough energy and strength to serve others by taking care of them—which is my passion in life. The routine encourages me to get out of bed and get my body in motion since I have my phone charging on the other side of the room with its face down (meaning I can't just shut off the alarm and go back to snoozing). The alarm I've set up also doesn't have a snooze option, so I know that getting back in bed isn't an option and that I need to get my day started.

When I'm up, I start my morning by praying out loud. My prayers are worded so that I say what I'm grateful for first, which starts my day with a thankful heart. I believe in God and thank Him for all that He's blessed me with in my life. For anyone who doesn't believe in God, I still think that starting your day off by saying what you're grateful for out loud will start your day on the best note possible. By saying it aloud, you hear it for yourself, and it sinks into your mind so that you hold a positive perspective from the earliest moments of your day. Raising your vibrational energy using prayer, your mind, or a journal to express gratitude is a very healthy way to start the day.

ACTION STEP

Take a few minutes to write down the things you're grateful for in a journal. The list can be long or short, and you can have a lot of detail or very little. But direct your conscious mind to what you're grateful for, for at least a few minutes. Say it out loud if you would like to. Better yet, tell the person you're thankful towards, that you're grateful for them, and why you are. This will provide a positive bonding experience that can make both your day and theirs. So, in keeping it simple, ask yourself, "what am I grateful for today?" Do this in the morning and at night, and you'll nurture a healthy mindset that will pull you up on a continuous basis.

7

POSITIVE AFFIRMATIONS

"Instead of worrying about what you cannot control, shift your energy to what you can create."

— ROY T. BENNETT

WHO DO YOU WANT TO BE?

Affirmations are things you say with the intention of making them appear true or bringing them into existence. Positive affirmations are used with the purpose of bringing the mind into a better state by focusing on things that bring happiness and success. Using them can change the direction of your life upwards, and you can have a better impact on the people and situations you face.

The statements made are repeated over and over with the purpose of manifesting them. The psychological effect is that we make ourselves believe something will come true or is possible, thus making us more driven to bring it into reality. By stating positive affirmations, we replace old and negative neural pathways with new ones that attempt to solve things and face situations in a more direct and optimistic nature. To achieve the best results with positive affirmations, we need to be persistent and consistent with our use.

HOW TO USE POSITIVE AFFIRMATIONS

First, you have to pick a phrase or phrases that you're going to affirm. Choose one that's relevant to an area in which you're negative or where you're not doing too great. The affirmation needs to be positive, and it needs to have the intention of lifting you up in that area where you're not doing too well. Say it aloud daily or write it down so that it sinks in and you get your mind thinking about that concept.

You can move around while you're saying it to add motion as a different technique to base the affirmation in reality. Activities could include gestures, specific movements, walking around, or exercising. You can add further stimuli like smells (for example, from scented candles) so that you associate that stimulus with the affirmation you're making. Thus, every time you encounter that pleasant stimulus, you'll unconsciously be reminding yourself of the affirmation you used while in its presence.

Say your affirmations in the present tense, as if what you're affirming is busy happening. This focuses on your affirmation and contributes to the concept of it materializing. Keep the wording simple, and try to put emotion into what you say. You should feel it as if it's true. Don't use negative language because this focuses on the opposite of what you want to affirm. By stating that you're avoiding some condition, you're only making it stronger (such as "I don't want to be fat," serving to focus your affirmation on the fact that you believe you're already fat.) Keep the wording positively phrased.

When you can, add specifics and details to what you're saying. This will make the affirmation more effective. So if you want to be rich, it might be helpful for you to specify, "I have 2 million dollars in my bank account." So long as the specifics don't make the wording too complicated, you can add the detail you thought of. To make your affirmation more powerful, visualize what you're saying with all the specifics possible. Having all the perceptions of the event materializing in your mind will help the affirmation sink better into your subconscious.

I use positive affirmations in my life by strategically placing them in places I will see throughout the day, consciously or subconsciously. I have them on two notecards taped to my bathroom mirror, the background of my phone, and on sticky notes at my computer at work. Some examples of the affirmations that I use are as follows:

1. A peaceful mind is a strong mind.
2. Who are you when no one is watching?
3. The one who listens understands.
4. What are you grateful for today?
5. My value comes from who I am, not from what I do.
6. Anything that happens to me today is in my best interest and is an opportunity to learn and grow.
7. Don't let the winds of the world blow out the fire of your soul.
8. Seek Clarity, Generate Energy, Raise Necessity, Increase Productivity, Develop Influence, Demonstrate Courage.

These phrases are gentle reminders from numerous books I have read throughout the years and have stuck with me. I change them periodically, but they continue to bring me new perspectives as I grow older. They always help to clear my mind and provide me with inspiration and motivation to be the best version of myself.

HOW CAN POSITIVE AFFIRMATIONS BE USED FOR PAIN RELIEF?

You can cause pain in your body to relieve when you keep your mindset positive. Your perception of the pain will reduce, and the cause of the pain will often start healing or improving faster than before. To be effective, you need to use affirmations repetitively for this purpose; it can't be a once-off thing. The need for repetition is due to neuroplasticity requiring a new neural process to be used multiple times before it replaces an old one. The old ones (that lead you to think in terms that make the pain more prominent) have resilience and need some time before they are fully disestablished.

Some positive affirmations that are useful for pain-related conditions include:

- I have strong and healthy joints
- I'm experiencing a pain release
- My (body part that's affected) feels relaxed
- I can move my body easily
- My body provides the strength and support I need
- I have a reliable body that feels good

The above affirmations are worded so that you're not focusing on pain but on comfort, relaxation, and strength. Many affirmations that you find on the internet about pain expressly say, "don't feel pain," which just puts your attention back on feeling it. Instead, use words that describe conditions opposite to pain or at variance with it. Some terms you should consider are painless, comfortable, vital, strong, capable, powerful, potent, and relaxed.

HOW CAN POSITIVE AFFIRMATIONS BE USED FOR STRESS AND ANXIETY?

Affirmations can be used to have a calming effect on your mind, thus relaxing it when you're going through periods of stress or anxiety. You can use the affirmations directly on the subject of anxiety, bringing a reality into play of you being more at ease. Or, you can use your affirmations on other subjects and feel the relaxation that naturally comes with it. Positive affirmations slowly change the way we think by altering the synapses in our neural pathways. In addition to using affirmations to positively affect your mind, use positive self-talk throughout your day to uplift you emotionally.

To overcome anxiety, you'll first need to determine what your current mindset is. See in what areas you're feeling anxious or negative. Those are the areas on which to focus to become more positive. Make a firm decision that those areas will change and that you will make definitive progress in them. When you think of a negative thought relating to that area of your life, think of one or more positive thoughts following this to counteract the negativity.

When you know that a stressful experience is going to come up, such as a job interview, then make positive affirmations about it beforehand. Go into the interview with as realistically optimistic of a mindset as you can. Repeat your affirmations to yourself in your mind if you get stressed during the interview. If you feel stressed after the experience and while doing follow-ups, don't hesitate to repeat the positive affirmations to yourself.

When you make the affirmations, if you're realistically optimistic, you're more likely to be able to achieve what you set your mind to. And you're more likely to do it with lower levels of anxiety. Nothing creates stress on the mind, like expecting the impossible. When you don't achieve the impossible after you'd forced yourself to think you would, you end up feeling down and depressed about it. To avoid all of this, be positive but realistically so.

A few affirmations that you might want to use to gain more control over stress levels include:

- I feel safe
- I confidently handle situations that I need to face
- The troubles I faced have become a stepping stone on my path to success
- This situation is neither good nor bad, and it's something for me to handle routinely
- The obstacle I just faced is now in the past

When you make your affirmations, take it a step further. Put your affirmations into action by seeing how you can implement a positive mindset in your life. Cement positivity in with healthy action.

ACTION STEP

Set aside about half an hour so that you can complete this action step from start to end. Get yourself a spot where you won't be bothered, then lightly introspect. You're looking for thought patterns you're using that are sabotaging you, whether directly or indirectly. See what the thought patterns are and what they pertain to, then work out an affirmation that counteracts it. You might need to reword it a few times until you have really catchy wording that strikes a chord with you. Say it out loud to yourself at several points of the day, and make little notes all over the place that will remind you of your affirmation. This could be sticky notes, appropriately worded reminders or alarms on your phone, notes at the top of your daily planner, or any number of other places. Do this continually for weeks on end, changing the wording of your affirmation if the initial one starts becoming dull. You'll notice how it picks you up after a while.

8

MOVEMENT

"Consciousness is only possible through change; change is only possible through movement."

— ALDOUS HUXLEY

HOW CAN YOU PRIORITIZE MORE MOVEMENT?

Movement is medicine, and we must prioritize it in our daily routines. Exercise is something that we all know has a lot of benefits. Undoubtedly, without any form of physical activity or exercise, we would waste away physically and be incapable of sustaining our bodies. On the flip side, there's adequate exercise or exercise that's more than good enough. In these cases, exercise can be one of the best things for our physical, chemical, and emotional health.

When you exercise, you improve your brain's health and overall functioning. This increases the quality and speed of your thinking, learning, and judgment. Not to mention that when you exercise, your brain releases pleasure-giving hormones that pull you up from negative emotions so that you enjoy yourself in the present. This is why exercise is promoted as a healthy coping mechanism—you get your "high," but without the after-effects of drugs and alcohol.

Your overall body strength is increased from exercising, particularly your muscles, joints, and bones. The chemical processes in your body function better, and it will feel more comfortable from added flexibility and endurance. Your heart, in particular, is a muscle that improves in strength when you exercise routinely. This lowers your risk of exposure to heart diseases while contributing to lower blood pressure and healthier cholesterol levels.

You lower your risk of type two diabetes by keeping physically active. Excess calories, sugar, and fat are burned off, and hormones or chemicals that process your food are released as they should be. This, in turn, helps with weight management, which affects us physically and in terms of our self-image. Exercise doesn't only lower the risk of heart disease and diabetes but also several types of cancers. Large quantities of research haven't been done yet, but the results are promising so far.

BENEFITS OF EXERCISE FOR PAIN RELIEF

When you exercise, you can overcome short periods of pain, as well as reduce chronic pain levels (pain lasting longer than three months). This happens with low, dull aches as well as sharp, intense pain sensations. When we experience chronic pain, it affects us physically because we don't want to get up and be active but would rather remain inactive to not aggravate it more. It affects us emotionally because we get frustrated with the pain persisting despite our best efforts at eradicating it. It also affects us mentally because our minds are preoccupied with the sensations we're feeling, so we can't put all of our attention on the tasks that demand our attention. Often, this can lead to mental health concerns such as depression or anxiety.

It might seem counterintuitive when you're sitting there with a sore leg or back that flares up each time you move, but getting physically active is a solution to the situation. It acts to reduce current pain and, in the long run, functions as a preventative measure to pain. This is partly because of the strengthened muscles and bones that you get when routinely exercising. It's also because of the lower levels of fatigue you experience from the higher quality of sleep and the chemicals that are released from the brain throughout the body. Another reason is that when you exercise, the pain signals that travel through your nerves are normalized and stop working in dysfunctional ways. With pain signals traveling properly, pain-inhibition chemicals are released more regularly, and tissue-healing chemicals are issued as they should be.

BENEFITS OF EXERCISE FOR STRESS AND ANXIETY

Exercise lowers your levels of short-term anxiety. The instant twinges of anxiety you feel when a stressful situation comes up are easier to manage and aren't as intense for long. The same applies to bouts of depression and to long-term anxiety. This is largely because of improved sleep and a better mood that accompanies getting your body in motion to burn energy and increase strength. It acts to ease the symptoms of anxiety and depression, as well as lowering the chances of it recurring.

When you exercise, endorphins are released, resulting in an improved perception of pleasure. You feel a heightened sense of well-being, naturally resulting in less worrying and negative thoughts. Your level of self-confidence and self-image also rise, thereby lowering the chances of someone bringing you down with nastiness or stress-producing requests. With your improved level of ease regarding yourself, interacting with others is more comfortable, which brings about a lower sense of social anxiety. Further, exercise often leads to social interaction in relaxed settings (such as chatting with joggers in the street), thereby introducing pleasant socialization into your daily life.

WALKING OUTSIDE

This is one of the exercises that I enjoy the most. This shouldn't be surprising coming from a chiropractor, but you should prioritize it in your daily routine. I also advise that you have a mobility routine, like yoga, to start your day every day and a stretching routine to wind down at the end of the day. A body in motion stays in motion. You are only blessed with one body, and you must take care of it.

You may want to do other physical activities every day, but I'm not going to tell you which ones. If you find something you enjoy, then you'll keep on doing it, but if you're instructed to do something you don't enjoy, then you're going to do it for a while and stop. For instance, I love lifting weights for the benefits resistance training provides, so I've kept on doing it as part of my exercise plan for the rest of my life. When you've found something you enjoy, incorporate it into your daily routine and run with it. In the meantime, walking is something that's pleasant for most of us and can be done as a physical activity (both as a main activity and as an auxiliary to other exercises).

When I say walking, I'm referring to walking outside. Walking outside allows you to connect with nature and will provide you with the grounding you need for a calm and happy mindset. Breathe in fresh air while you walk and soak up the sunlight. Listen to the sounds of the birds and the rustling of the leaves. Smell the flowers as you walk by them and feel the temperature of the breeze on your skin. Walking on a treadmill doesn't provide you with all of this.

Walking outside allows you to embrace the use of your senses. It raises your consciousness of the world, making it a great way to start the day with an alert mindset. With all the pleasure that comes with connecting to nature while you walk, you have all the motivation you need to keep walking incorporated into your regular exercise routine.

One of the benefits of routine walks outside is that it improves your mood. Endorphins get released, and you feel good and lower your pain and stress. Further, you increase your vitamin D intake levels by exposing your body to the sun, and when you walk outside for a few minutes to an hour a day, you can take in healthy levels of sunlight. Vitamin D is a mood enhancer, which is one reason why people who are always inside or who live in countries with low sun levels are more likely to feel depressed. In addition to better vitamin D intake and the release of endorphins, walking outside also releases serotonin, which gives you a feeling of well-being and lowers anxiety and depression levels.

Walking outside for half an hour per day, five days a week, significantly reduces the risk for coronary artery disease, other cardiovascular conditions, and strokes. Other diseases (including chronic ones and some cancers) are also less likely to affect those who regularly walk than those who don't. Further, it's a good way of keeping obesity and weight-related conditions at bay. It keeps excessive fat at bay by releasing the hormone irisin while you exercise, as well as afterward.

You will notice that you also function better mentally when you walk often. This may include better memory, decision-making, and creativity. For those of us that like doing creative activities, this is the perfect exercise to do when you're running into a creative blockage. With a combination of improved physical and mental health conditions from walking regularly (especially if it's between four and eight thousand steps per day), you're also likely to increase your longevity.

Other than keeping you healthy and decreasing the risks you face over the course of your life, walking outside is also an excellent way to keep your family bonds strong. I go for a walk outside (weather permitting) with my daughter and our dog after dinner for 15 minutes to an hour. It ensures that our digestion functions are at their best and that our blood sugar levels stay healthy. Further, it's an excellent way for her to have fun while I enjoy the happiness that comes with being a present father.

ACTION STEP

Build a walk into your daily routine. This could be when you first wake up, on your lunch break, or after dinner. A 15 to 30-minute walk is a good length. It'll aid your digestion and control your energy levels; who wants energy spikes and crashes, after all? To make the walk an even better experience, incorporate your family when you can or a friend or two. It's an excellent time to bond socially and a good way to ensure all of you keep healthy.

9

BREATHWORK

"Conscious breathing is the best antidote to stress, anxiety, and depression."

— AMIT RAY

CAN YOU VISUALIZE YOUR BREATH?

Breathwork is when you use conscious breathing techniques to increase the intake of oxygen into your body and the flow of toxins out of your body. The purpose is to affect a smooth interchange of clean air and waste with maximum ease. I often visualize my breath coming in through my nose and filling my lungs, then exiting my body and deflating my lungs. I imagine this as a rhythmic circle flowing in and out of my body. When you can do this, you nourish your body, mind, and spirit.

Deep Breathing

Deep breathing is the practice of intentionally taking in deep breaths so that your lungs are as full of air as possible. It's an exercise that improves the strength of your breathing muscles and organs while training them to function better on a day-to-day basis. One of the main benefits of doing this type of breathing as a regular exercise is that it exercises your diaphragm to expand and contract up and down better. As a result, you'll lower your blood pressure and stress levels, making yourself feel calmer and centered.

Nasal Breathing

When you breathe through your mouth, you're bringing in particles without filtration. This makes it easier for bacteria to enter your body. When you breathe through your nose, the hairs (cilia) filter out dust and other particles, meaning the air you breathe in is cleaner and better for your body. The temperature of the air is also improved for your lungs' use because your nose and nasal passage warms it and allows moisture levels to be optimized. Further, breathing through your nose rather than your mouth improves oxygen circulation in your body by widening your blood vessels by releasing nitric acid.

It might be challenging to breathe comfortably using your nose if you've developed a habit of using your mouth some or all of the time. To regain the habit of nasal breathing, try belly breathing, breath of fire, and alternate nostril breathing (all of which are described below).

Some of the main benefits of using nasal breathing include the following:

- better lung capacity
- better oxygen flow in your bloodstream
- lower intake of dust, pollen, and other air-borne particles
- slower breathing, which has a calming effect
- a stronger diaphragm
- less coughing from particles and spit flowing into your lungs
- the air you breathe having appropriate humidity and warmth levels
- less snoring
- lower risk of sleep apnea

Breath Awareness

Breath awareness is simply the practice of noticing that you're breathing and how you're breathing. You're not altering your breath in any way, and you're not doing any sort of exercise with your respiratory system. When you pay attention to your breathing for a while, being mindful of things like the sound of the air going in and out, the flow of air, how fast you're breathing, and how deep your breaths are, you'll see how your breathing can be improved. In the process, you'll activate your parasympathetic nervous system, creating a sense of calm.

Breath-Based Meditation

Focusing on your breathing is one of the most common aspects of meditation. There are multiple techniques that center around the flow of air in and out of your body and the way you breathe. It's particularly effective at keeping you in the present moment because you're focusing on a process that continually happens. When doing breath-based meditation, you're not doing breathwork as such because you're simply noting your breathing rather than trying to make it deeper.

BENEFITS

Breathwork is an effective tool for calming down and elevating your mood. It slows the body into normal functioning, so you're not operating in a fight-or-flight mode. You'll reduce the intensity of trauma and PTSD when you use breathwork, as well as anxiety and depression. It's good at healing emotional wounds faster and improving our outlook on life. When someone has a problem with addiction, breathwork can effectively ease their reliance on substances or actions they're addicted to.

Part of the reason why it provides so many benefits is that breathwork improves your circulation, blood pressure, and pH level. Chemical processes in your body happen as they should, and there's a better release of toxins generated in the process. Your immune system is positively affected, resulting in a lower risk of illness. Your muscle tone can develop better, and pain levels will be managed better.

Breathing correctly will improve your digestion and sleep, resulting in more sustained energy levels. With good energy levels and a vital body, you'll find it easier to feel happy and alert.

CAN BREATHWORK BE USED FOR PAIN RELIEF?

With the activation of the parasympathetic nervous system, the fight-or-flight response calms down. Your heart rate and blood pressure drop, and pleasure hormones are released. Fears are lowered, and your expectation of an impending threat vanishes when this is unfounded. You regain good blood flow, and your muscles relax, allowing your body to restore oxygen saturation and appropriate chemical processes. So the answer is most emphatically, "yes, breathwork can be used for pain relief."

Coupling breathwork with creative visualization and some forms of meditation can further enhance your pain management. With visualization of your pain-inducing body part(s) in optimal condition and the calmness brought about by deep breathing, you'll be contributing to the improvement of your body's pain management and healing. The process of visualization coupled with meditation and breathwork can speed up the alteration of neural pathways from those that induce body pain.

CAN BREATHWORK BE USED FOR STRESS AND ANXIETY?

The reduction of your anxiety as a result of breathwork is a result of many physical changes that take place. This includes a slower heart rate, muscles becoming less tense, lower blood pressure, more nitric acid for better blood flow and oxygen saturation, and a decrease in your metabolism. The relaxation in question doesn't result in you being lulled into a state of sleepiness. It results in your body being relaxed but your mind becoming more focused and calm.

Using 20 to 30 minutes of abdominal breathing daily is one of the most effective techniques for reducing anxiety and stress. It saturates your body and brain with oxygen and activates the parasympathetic nervous system. You remain connected to your body throughout the process and lose connection with the worries or distractions flying around your head.

Diaphragmatic breathing is a good tool for chronic pain management. Place a hand on your belly and a hand on your chest, feeling how they move when you breathe in and out.

When you use your diaphragm for breathing, you'll notice that your belly rises and falls with each breath. Take ten deep breaths like this to calm the nerves and make you feel ready to continue with the day.

Box breathing (also called square breathing) is a deep breathing method that's great for soothing your nervous system. You sit or lie down with a hand on your chest and a hand on your belly. If you're sitting, keep your back straight and your feet flat on the floor. Breathe normally for a bit, then start taking deep breaths. If you need to, push out your tummy while you're learning how to breathe deeply. You'll know that you're truly breathing deeply when your upper back moves against the chair or surface you're against. Breathe in for four seconds, hold for four, breathe out for four, and hold for four. Repeat this until you feel calm. Counting is a good distraction from your thoughts, making this breathing technique faster than others in terms of relaxing you.

The 4-7-8 breathing is similar to box breathing, but you breathe in for four seconds, hold for seven, then breathe out for eight. This is a type of rhythmic breathing that practices your lung-emptying function. It's particularly effective for improving sleep quality by getting your body into a calm, rhythmic state.

Another technique you can use for stress is alternate nostril breathing (which is also an excellent technique to get yourself used to daily nasal breathing). Close your right nostril with your right thumb and breathe in using your left nostril. Hold your breath, remove your thumb from the right nostril, and close the left with your left thumb. Once complete, breathe out through your right nostril. Then breathe in with the right nostril, swap to close the right nostril, then breathe out through the left. Continue alternating like this so that you're alternately breathing in and out in a balanced fashion. Continue this until you feel calmer.

BEST BREATHWORK TECHNIQUES FOR BEGINNERS

Some of the easier breathwork techniques were covered above in the breathwork for anxiety section. A few other simple techniques follow here that you can use for everyday breathing enhancement.

Pursed lip breathing is used to slow the breath and is often used by individuals with asthma or conditions that block their lung functioning. To do it:

1. Sit comfortably, then relax your back, neck, and shoulders.
2. Inhale with your mouth closed for two seconds, then purse your lips so that you can exhale out of them. The exhalation should last for about four seconds.
3. Continue doing this until your body feels at ease.

Deep abdominal breathing is similar to deep breathing but with the addition of visualization. While breathing deeply so that your lungs fill to total capacity, visualize your whole body filling with air in your mind's eye. Once a full breath has been achieved, breathe out in a relaxed way. Do this over and over until your body feels unwound.

The breath of fire technique is more advanced and can be attempted once you're comfortable with the preceding techniques. To do it:

1. Breathe in with your abdomen relaxed. There shouldn't be tension in your abdominal muscles at all while you're breathing in.
2. Once you've finished inhaling, push the air out with force using your abdominal muscles.
3. Repeat this until you manage to do it without much difficulty.

An advanced technique that you might have heard of is holotropic breathing. Don't use this technique without a professional. It's a technique in which you breathe in and out without pause, similar to the way you would when hyperventilating. This is done with a breathing partner to make sure that you don't pass out and get hurt or otherwise do yourself harm. When done correctly, you enter a state of altered consciousness (almost as if you had taken a drug like LSD), which allows you to influence your mental and emotional state in predetermined ways. This technique has been rewarding for many people, but avoid it as a beginner and make sure that you have a trained breathing partner if you do attempt it.

PERSONAL NOTES

Your breathing influences your whole body and directly affects your health. It is arguably the most important part of health, going above healthy eating and exercise. You regulate your nervous system with it and keep yourself stable through many ups and downs using it. It's something you can use no matter what you're stressed about, whether it be money, your job, health, conflicts at home, or any number of other things. You might not be able to control things in your life, but you can control your breath. "Working" your breath properly prepares you for the things you need to face.

When we get upset with someone, we're often told to "take ten deep breaths." Why? When you breathe consciously, you calm your nervous system and enter a parasympathetic state. If you get tired while exercising, you control your breathing to deliver more oxygen to your brain and muscles. Exerting yourself requires more oxygen, so breathe to make that available.

Even calming practices like meditation use breathing as their primary focus in many cases. Guided meditation specifically mentions breathing to help you clear the stresses of the day out of your mind. They require that you note the air going in as your lungs expand and your belly flattening out as you exhale. Often you're also asked to visualize the air going in and out.

Breathwork is one of my favorite pain management techniques to discuss with clients. I make sure they understand the importance of breathwork, and I hope that now you do too. When it comes to breathing, there are two things I'm particularly passionate about. One is nasal breathing, and the other is my favorite breathwork technique.

I have been focusing on nasal breathing for about two years after reading *Breath* by James Nestor. Using nasal breathing when I sleep improves the quality of my sleep, decreases my snoring (much to the relief of my wife), gives me more energy throughout the day, and has even stopped me from needing to get up to pee in the middle of the night. That's right. Nasal breathing helps decrease the frequency of urination. I've listed a research article at the end of the book if you want to look more into this. I use Breathe Right™ Nasal Strips and mouth tape to achieve these improvements.

My favorite breathwork technique is belly breathing (also known as diaphragmatic breathing or abdominal breathing). Although I described it above, I want to add a note. When a patient asks me, "What's the best exercise to help strengthen my core?" My answer is "belly breathing." It works by using your muscles to force your diaphragm to move as you breathe in, allowing the lungs to fill up with more air. If you are intentional with this technique and practice it consistently, you will see your quality of life improve.

ACTION STEP

Use diaphragmatic breathing every morning. Take 33 full breaths each time, breathing in and out through your nose. For added benefit, place one hand on your heart and the other on your belly. Repeat the phrase, "I love you. I am listening" to yourself. This reiterates your love for yourself and your ability to listen to your body's needs. Do this for a month and see what benefits you experience. Note them down and acknowledge the positive change it's made. Continue with daily diaphragmatic breathing, keeping your mind and body in excellent condition.

MEDITATION

> *"If you are quiet enough, you will hear the flow of the universe. You will feel its rhythm. Go with this flow. Happiness lies ahead. Mediation is key."*
>
> — BUDDHA

IS MEDITATION THE KEY TO PEACE?

Meditation is a method of focusing and clearing the mind with the purpose of generating benefits for your mind and soul. It's a practice that's thousands of years old and has been an important practice in multiple religions and philosophies (such as

Christianity, Buddhism, and Taoism). Sometimes other practices are incorporated into it, like repeating a mantra or sound, visualizing things, breathwork, and movement techniques. One of the primary purposes behind it is to increase your ability to focus, whether this is focusing your mind on your body or the environment, something in your mind like an idea or question, or a higher power such as a deity or God. Prayer is considered to be a type of meditation, particularly when practiced in a contemplative way.

Mindfulness is an essential element of meditation. You'll find it easier to remain in the present and not veer off into the past, the future, or your mind as an escape. Using the sensation your body feels internally as you're meditating is one way of incorporating mindfulness into it, while focusing on the stimuli in your environment is another. This positively affects your brain and mental health by increasing the density of your neural network in areas pertaining to your senses, thinking and concentration, and processing of emotions.

Meditation can be done alone, or it can be done in groups. When done in groups, it's usually done with the help of a teacher who issues gentle instructions and incorporates guided imagery. Group meditation is often done as part of counseling interventions and addiction recovery.

STRESS, ANXIETY, AND MEDITATION

One of the primary purposes behind meditation is to reduce stress and anxiety. It's been known to help people with anxiety disorders, depression, and post-traumatic stress disorder. It works by breaking through the jumbled thoughts of the mind and making it less crowded. Your attention gets moved from something stressful to something relaxing, and you get the opportunity to refocus on positive things. Emotional and physical benefits from mediation include:

- higher patience and tolerance
- managing your triggers better
- boosting creativity
- less negative thinking
- present-orientation
- improved stress management
- gaining new perspectives and ways of thinking
- higher self-awareness

ELEMENTS OF MEDITATION

Meditation has five main elements: focused attention, a comfortable position, an open attitude, relaxed breathing, and a quiet setting.

Focused attention is generated by keeping your observation abilities directed at a specific thing or condition. This could be an object (such as a trophy), your body (by doing self-scanning, for instance), a health condition you want (such as joints that move comfortably), or any number of other things.

A comfortable position could be sitting, lying down, standing, posing, stretching, or even walking around. Sitting and lying down are the easiest to do when you're starting out with meditation because it's easier to focus. When sitting, keeping a good posture helps a lot.

Having an open attitude is essential because a closed mind will result in an unwillingness to be there and observe comfortably. It would be best if you were willing to have your thoughts come up without judging them, followed by lightly acknowledging them and continuing with your meditation. You will have thoughts that come up about all sorts of things. If you get upset with yourself about not having your mind clear, you're never going to get to the point of attaining calm through meditation. To achieve that calm, accept that thoughts will come up and don't get wrapped up in them when they do.

Relaxed breathing is both necessary for the physical benefits of meditation and to give yourself something to focus on when you get distracted. Breathing is sometimes altered so that you can practice breathwork while doing meditation. Other times, you merely use breath awareness to observe your breathing as it normally happens.

The final requirement, at least at first, is a quiet setting. However, when you have more experience meditating, there's no problem with meditating in the most stressful situations. But it remains easiest to do it in a distraction-free environment, where your focus can stay on yourself and what you're doing.

MEDITATION AND PAIN RELIEF

The normal solution for pain in pharmacology, particularly with severe or chronic pain, is opioids. While these are effective, the problem is that they can lead to addiction. Mindfulness meditation can bypass the opioid receptors in the brain, providing pain relief without the need for drugs. Neural pathways in the brain can be "rewired" so that old patterns that induce pain or prevent proper functioning of your pain-management systems and chemicals are ignored in favor of ones that allow proper functioning.

PERSONAL TAKE ON MEDITATION

Our brains can feel overwhelmed by all of the thoughts, news, and information that we receive on a daily basis. This can be similar to a computer running too many programs at once. Meditation is the perfect way to make our brains feel less overwhelmed by all the programs running simultaneously. It reboots our minds so that we can look at things from a fresh perspective. It's a healthy habit that makes us happier and helps us live more vibrantly. We enter a parasympathetic state and handle stressful situations more calmly. We should do it daily to gain the maximum benefits from this amazing art.

My favorite meditation method is lying on my back on my shakti mat for ten minutes before bed. As a chiropractor, I recommend a shakti mat (also called an acupressure mat) to all my patients. It helps to decrease stress, reduces muscle tension, increases blood flow, and brings attention and awareness to the 6000+ acupressure points being stimulated while you lie down. I often have patients tell me they experience an emotional benefit just as much as a physical one. I highly recommend it if you've never used a shakti mat.

BENEFITS OF MEDITATION

The mental benefits available from meditation are pretty dramatic. It improves your level of problem-solving. How you think is enhanced by having a clearer mind that's easier to focus. With your clearer mind, it's also easier to confront emotional problems and process negative feelings. Higher levels of joy are a natural reaction to having your emotional strain lightened. With your positive emotions rising to the surface, it's easier to be kind-hearted towards others and to make them feel comfortable around you. In other words, your social environment can become a more pleasant one.

Your body is also impacted positively with better sleep, healthier blood pressure, and proper heart functioning. Not having the fight or flight reaction in continuous stimulation allows your body to operate at a normal level, which is much better for you in the long run.

ACTION STEP

Get yourself comfortable by sitting and crossing your legs with your back in a natural curve of good posture. Do this while sitting on a pillow for the best relaxation. Bring yourself to the present by noticing the position your legs are in and how it feels. Drop your hands onto the top of your legs in a comfortable position. Gently bring your chin down so that it's in a comfortable position, with your head facing down slightly. Bring your eyes to a close.

Notice your breathing and bring yourself into the present moment. Notice your breath flowing in and going out. Keep focusing on it and let your thoughts drift away. If your mind goes to something, acknowledge that your attention went to something else, and then (without being forceful or upset with yourself) bring your attention back to your breathing. Your mind will probably wander multiple times within the first few minutes. Don't judge yourself when this happens; just bring your attention back to the flow of air going in and out.

If you hear things in your surroundings or sense some other stimuli (like a smell or a sensation), observe it with acceptance. Don't try to change anything. Just accept your body, thoughts, and surroundings as they are. All the while, bring your attention back to your breathing every time it drifts, just noticing it comfortably. When you feel like you've reached a comfortable point in your meditation session, bring yourself back to your present and open your eyes. Do a brief inventory of how you feel and a comparison with how you felt before your session.

Meditation doesn't have to be complicated to be effective. You can find moments throughout the day when you do straightforward meditation techniques. You can get into a meditative state while walking, cleaning, painting, crafting, reading, coloring, gardening, writing, or any number of other daily actions. So long as they ease your mind, bring you to the present moment, and keep you in a relaxed state. If they bring you to a state of consciously living in the present and connecting your body and mind for calmness and clarity, then they should be used for precisely that. Prioritize your life and your mind by deciding on a meditation practice for you and prioritizing it as part of your daily routine. A peaceful mind is a strong mind. A strong mind is a healthy mind.

CONCLUSION

The quality of your life is determined by the quality of your questions. I started each chapter in this book with a question to consider for each topic. When you are feeling pain, stress, or anxiety, go back to these questions and work through the answers. The answers have the ability to change your perspective and transform your life.

This book covered three main areas of your living where you can directly impact your health. These are your mind and the thoughts you have, the words you use, and the actions you take to find healing and peace in your life. The tools included a range of mindfulness techniques, strategies to control your subconscious mind and better understand your ego, the philosophy of Stoicism (and overcoming the fear of death), creative visualization, expressing gratitude, positive affirmations, movement and exercise, breathwork, and meditation.

You now have the tools you need to bring anxiety, stress, and pain under your own control. These methods are natural and don't require that you put any artificial chemicals into your body. You're utilizing what you already have—your mind, your body, and the environment. Use the information you've learned in this book to make your life better. Only benefits await.

I hope you've enjoyed the book and learned something that you can take with you for the rest of your life. My biggest goal in publishing it is to give you the confidence to use the information provided to help you live a healthier, happier, and higher quality of life. I would really love your honest feedback and would appreciate a review on Amazon or whatever platform you used to get the book. I know this book can help a lot of people, and a review can help others better understand what they can gain from it.

Thank you from the bottom of my heart for reading. I appreciate you. If you would like to connect on social media, feel free to reach out via Instagram @DrJordanBurns.

In Health,

Jordan

REFERENCES

Amy Spies. (n.d.). *About Amy*. Retrieved December 4, 2022, from https://www.amyspies.com/about#bio

Alexander, R. (2010, July 27). What are the limitations of your ego mind? *Psychology Today*. https://www.psychologytoday.com/us/blog/the-wise-open-mind/201007/what-are-the-limitations-your-ego-mind

Altruism in Medicine Institute. (2017). *Accepting and embracing fear with Dr. Barry Kerzin* [Video]. In YouTube. https://www.youtube.com/watch?v=rOP8TlTbaIQ

Andrus, J. L. F. (2017, November 15). *Breathing techniques for natural pain relief*. Orthopaedic and Spine Center. https://www.osc-ortho.com/blog/breathing-techniques-for-natural-pain-relief/#:~:text=A%20good%20pace%20is%204,and%20deflating%20as%20you%20breathe

Aperture. (2021). *Stoicism: Becoming undefeatable* [Video]. In YouTube. https://www.youtube.com/watch?v=EFkyxzJtiv4

Augustyn, A. (2021). Ego. *Encyclopedia Britannica*. https://www.britannica.com/topic/ego-philosophy-and-psychology

Baikie, K. A., & Wilhelm, K. (2005). Emotional and physical health benefits of expressive writing. *Advances in Psychiatric Treatment*, 11(5), 338–346. Cambridge Core. https://doi.org/10.1192/apt.11.5.338

Belfer, I., & Shurtleff, D. (Eds.). (2022, February). *Qigong: What you need to know*. National Center for Complementary and Integrative Health. https://www.nccih.nih.gov/health/qigong-what-you-need-to-know

Benefits of physical activity. (2022, June 16). Centers for Disease Control and Prevention. https://www.cdc.gov/physicalactivity/basics/pa-health/index.htm#:~:text=Being-physically-active-can-improve-activity-gain-some-health-benefits

Bennett, R. T. (2016, February 26). *The Light in the Heart Quotes*. GoodReads. https://www.goodreads.com/work/quotes/49604402

Blount, A. (2021, July 28). Ways to change a habit (J. Jelinek, Ed.). *Psych Central*. https://psychcentral.com/health/steps-to-changing-a-bad-habit#allow-slip-ups

Boag, S. (2017). Splitting (Defense mechanism). In V. Zeigler-Hill & T. Shackelford (Eds.), *Encyclopedia of Personality and Individual Differences* (pp. 1–4). Springer. https://doi.org/10.1007/978-3-319-28099-8_1427-1

Breath awareness: A powerful tool to bridge the body and mind. (n.d.). Physio Dynamik. Retrieved December 12, 2022, from https://physiodynamik.com/en/breath-the-body-and-mind/#:~:text=Becoming%20aware%20of%20our%20breath,We%20call%20this%20breath%20awareness

Breath Guidance. (2019). *What is breathwork?* [Video]. In YouTube. https://www.youtube.com/watch?v=wC-BU1W_vNg

Breathwork for beginners: 5 ways to learn and practice it. (2021, October 17). Othership. https://www.othership.us/resources/breathwork-for-beginners

Brennan, D. (Ed.). (2021a, April 8). *What is box breathing?* WebMD. https://www.webmd.com/balance/what-is-box-breathing

Brennan, D. (Ed.). (2021b, June 28). *What is breathwork?* WebMD. https://www.webmd.com/balance/what-is-breathwork

Brennan, D. (Ed.). (2022, February 3). *What Is a victim mentality?* WebMD. https://www.webmd.com/mental-health/what-is-a-victim-mentality

Buccilli, D. (2021, March 13). *You give life to what you give energy to.* LinkedIn. https://www.linkedin.com/pulse/you-give-life-what-energy-danny-buccilli/

Cal y Mayor Galindo, P. (2021, April 30). *What is gratitude? 5 ways to be thankful.* BetterUp. https://www.betterup.com/blog/gratitude-definition-how-to-practice

Can expressing gratitude improve your mental, physical health? (2022, December 6). Mayo Clinic Health System. https://www.mayoclinichealthsystem.org/hometown-health/speaking-of-health/can-expressing-gratitude-improve-health#:~:text=Expressing%20gratitude%20is%20associated%20with,everyone%20would%20be%20taking%20it

Celestine, N. (2020, August 15). *What is mindful breathing? Exercises, scripts, and videos* (J. Nash, Ed.). Positive Psychology. https://positivepsychology.com/mindful-breathing/#:~:text=Practicing%20mindful%20breathing%20is%20gently,breath%20from%20moment%20to%20moment

Chan, A., Kohler, W., Tsai, S., Grigg-Damberger, M., Hairston, K. G., & Johnson, W. E. (2013, May 30). *5 Experts Answer: Is Lack of Sleep Bad for Health?* Live Science. https://www.livescience.com/35629-5-experts-answer-trouble-sleeping-health.html

Character development. (n.d.). *APA Dictionary of Psychology*. American Psychological Association. Retrieved November 30, 2022, from https://dictionary.apa.org/character-development

Chen, W. (2016, March 16). *Mindfulness meditation reduces pain, bypasses opioid receptors.* National Center for Complimentary and Integrative Health. https://www.nccih.nih.gov/research/blog/mindfulness-meditation-reduces-pain-bypasses-opioid-receptors

Cherry, K. (2022, September 22). *What is mindfulness meditation?* (S. Romanoff, Ed.). Verywell Mind. https://www.verywellmind.com/mindfulness-meditation-88369

Chick, N. (2013). *Metacognition.* Vanderbilt University Center for Teaching. https://cft.vanderbilt.edu/guides-sub-pages/metacognition/

Conditioning. (n.d.). Psychologist World. Retrieved December 8, 2022, from https://www.psychologistworld.com/memory/conditioning-intro

Cook, G., & Marchant, J. (2016, January 19). The science of healing thoughts. *Scientific American.* https://www.scientificamerican.com/article/the-science-of-healing-thoughts/

Coupland, M. (2018, November 26). *Deep breathing can reduce fear and lessen chronic pain.* Ascellus. https://ascellus.com/deep-breathing-can-reduce-chronic-pain/

Cuncic, A. (n.d.). *Holotropic breathwork benefits and risks* (S. Clark, Ed.). Verywell Mind. Retrieved December 12, 2022, from https://www.verywellmind.com/holotropic-breathwork-4175431

Daily Stoic. (2022). *What is momento mori? (Explained in 5 minutes)* [Video]. In YouTube. https://www.youtube.com/watch?v=Jbt6VGOYU3E

Davis, D. M., & Hayes, J. A. (2012). What are the benefits of mindfulness? A wealth of new research has explored this age-old practice. Here's a look at its benefits for both clients and psychologists. *CE Corner*, 43(7), 64. American Psychological Association. https://www.apa.org/monitor/2012/07-08/ce-corner#

Deep breathing and relaxation. (n.d.). The University of Toledo. Retrieved December 7, 2022, from https://www.utoledo.edu/studentaffairs/counseling/anxietytoolbox/breathingandrelaxation.html#:~:text=Deep%20breathing%20and%20relaxation%20activate

Dehydration. (2022, April 14). National Health Service Inform. https://www.nhsinform.scot/illnesses-and-conditions/nutritional/dehydration#:~:text=Dehydration%20can%20also%20lead%20to

Depression and anxiety: Exercise eases symptoms. (2017, September 27). Mayo Clinic. https://www.mayoclinic.org/diseases-conditions/depression/in-depth/depression-and-exercise/art-20046495

Dr. Haley Perlus on Peak Performance. (2016). *Dr. Haley Perlus on how to use imagery and visualization to heal an injury* [Video]. YouTube. https://www.youtube.com/watch?v=ARhqkxBHA-s

Expressive writing. (n.d.). Greater Good Science Center. Retrieved December 4, 2022, from https://ggia.berkeley.edu/practice/expressive_writing

Fit4D. (2017, August 8). *The neuroscience of behavior change.* StartUp Health. https://healthtransformer.co/the-neuroscience-of-behavior-change-bcb567fa83c1

Flarey, D. (2022, October 19). *What Is movement meditation?* American Institute of Health Care Professionals. https://aihcp.net/2012/10/17/what-is-movement-meditation/#:~:text=Movement%20meditation%20is%20not%20your

Giving thanks can make you happier. (2021, August 14). Harvard Health Publishing. https://www.health.harvard.edu/healthbeat/giving-thanks-can-make-you-happier#:~:text=Gratitude%20is%20a%20way%20for,instead%20of%20what%20they%20lack

Greater Good Science Center. (2010, April 15). *Jon Kabat-Zinn: What is mindfulness?* Greater Good. https://greatergood.berkeley.edu/topic/mindfulness/definition

Griffin, R. M. (2014, April 1). *10 health problems related to stress that you can fix* (J. Goldberg, Ed.). WebMD. https://www.webmd.com/balance/stress-management/features/10-fixable-stress-related-health-problems

Guided imagery for arthritis pain. (n.d.). Arthritis Foundation. Retrieved December 11, 2022, from https://www.arthritis.org/health-wellness/treatment/complementary-therapies/natural-therapies/guided-imagery-for-arthritis-pain

Hecht, M. (2020, September 4). *Meditating for chronic pain management* (D. Weatherspoon, Ed.). Healthline. https://www.healthline.com/health/meditation-for-chronic-pain

Ho, L. (n.d.). *How to change habits by using your subconscious mind.* Lifehack. Retrieved November 29, 2022, from https://www.lifehack.org/865931/change-habits

How to get what you want by training your subconscious. (2021, February 1). Positive Performance Training. https://www.positiveperformancetraining.com/blog/training-your-subconscious

How to set SMART goals. (n.d.). Brian Tracy International. https://www.briantracy.com/blog/personal-success/smart-goals/

Brian Tracy International. (n.d.). *The 80 20 rule – The Pareto principle.* https://www.briantracy.com/blog/personal-success/how-to-use-the-80-20-rule-pareto-principle/

Hypnotherapy. (n.d.). *Psychology Today.* Retrieved December 8, 2022, from https://www.psychologytoday.com/za/therapy-types/hypnotherapy

Interact with us: Trauma and positive outcomes. (2018, December 6). Intercommunity Action. https://intercommunityaction.org/interact-us-trauma-positive-outcomes/#:~:text=In%20contrast%2C%20many%20individuals%20who

Isaacs, N. (2008, October 21). Bring more mindfulness onto the mat. *Yoga Journal.* https://www.yogajournal.com/practice/yoga-sequences/peace-of-mind/

Itani, O. (2021, April 9). *The one question that should guide your daily life: "How do I want to be remembered?"* Omar Itani. https://www.omaritani.com/blog/how-do-you-want-to-be-remembered

Johns, J. (2022). False self. *International Diary of Psychoanalysis* (Cengage). Encyclopedia. https://www.encyclopedia.com/psychology/dictionaries-thesauruses-pictures-and-press-releases/false-self

Johnson, J. (2018, September 5). How to tell if stress is affecting your sleep. *Medical News Today.* https://www.medicalnewstoday.com/articles/322994#stress-and-sleep

Kim, & Hill. (2010, January 26). *Transform your habits by conditioning your brain.* Dr. Kim and Dr. Hil. https://www.authenticityassociates.com/transform-your-habits-by-conditioning-your-brain/

Levin, M. (2016, October 26). The 5 destructive voices in our heads: 6 powerful steps to erase your self-limiting. *Inc.Africa.* https://incafrica.com/library/marissa-levin-6-powerful-steps-to-rewrite-your-self-limiting-beliefs

Logos. (n.d.). Public Broadcasting Service. Retrieved December 10, 2022, from https://www.pbs.org/faithandreason/theogloss/logos-body.html

Long, C. (2021, August 30). *How the parasympathetic nervous system can lower stress.* Hospital for Special Surgery. https://www.hss.edu/article_parasympathetic-nervous-system.asp#:~:text=The%20parasympathetic%20nervous%20system%20is

Magnusson, K. R., & Brim, B. L. (2014). The aging brain. *Reference Module in Biomedical Sciences.* Science Direct. https://doi.org/10.1016/b978-0-12-801238-3.00158-6

McLeod, S. (2007). What is social psychology? Definition, theories & examples. *Simply Psychology.* www.simplypsychology.org/social-psychology.html

Meditation. (2022, May 22). Cleveland Clinic. https://my.clevelandclinic.org/health/articles/17906-meditation

Meditation and journaling: Combining practices to reflect your inner world. (n.d.). Kripalu Center for Yoga and Health. Retrieved December 4, 2022, from https://kripalu.org/resources/meditation-and-journaling-combining-practices-reflect-your-inner-world

Meditation: A simple, fast way to reduce stress. (2022, April 29). Mayo Clinic. https://www.mayoclinic.org/tests-procedures/meditation/in-depth/meditation/art-20045858

Metacognition. (n.d.). Teaching for Effective Learning. Retrieved November 27 C.E., from https://www.queensu.ca/teachingandlearning/modules/students/24_metacognition.html#:~:text=Metacognition%20is%20the%20process%20of

Metacognition. (2019). Cambridge Assessment International Education. chrome-extension://efaidnbmnnnibpcajpcglclefindmkaj/https://www.cambridgeinternational.org/Images/272307-metacognition.pdf

Miller, A. (n.d.). *10 ways to use sensory experiences to build mindfulness*. Happify. Retrieved December 5, 2022, from https://www.happify.com/hd/use-sensory-experiences-to-build-mindfulness/#:~:text=Researchers%20have%20found%20that%20mindfulness,%2C%20labeling%2C%20and%20letting%20go

Miller, M. (2017, August 29). *Pursue noble goals in the six seconds model of EQ*. Six Seconds. https://www.6seconds.org/2017/08/29/pursue-noble-goals/

Mindful Meditations. (2021). *Visualization for stress relief - Guided meditation* [Video]. YouTube. https://www.youtube.com/watch?v=WK99XAkxKyI&t=407s

Mindvalley. (2016). *Creative visualization for healing | Vishen Lakhiani* [Video]. YouTube. https://www.youtube.com/watch?v=88xWJsZM3D4

Mindvalley Talks. (2022). *Guided meditation: How to access altered states of mind | Vishen* [Video]. In YouTube. https://www.youtube.com/watch?v=cmgxNnVsILc&t=7s

Molitor, M. (2019, October 5). *The power of your brain | The 95-5% rule*. LinkedIn. https://www.linkedin.com/pulse/95-5-rule-michele-molitor-cpcc-pcc-rtt-c-hyp/?trk=portfolio_article-card_title

Moore, L. (n.d.). *Survival mode is killing you*. Mastermind Connect. Retrieved December 8, 2022, from https://mastermindconnect.com/blog/survival-mode-is-killing-you#:~:text=Survival%20mode%20is%20the%20short

Murphy, J. L., & Rafie, S. (2021, December 7). *5 exercises to ease chronic pain with gratitude*. Psychology Today. https://www.psychologytoday.com/us/blog/ease-pain/202112/5-exercises-ease-chronic-pain-gratitude

N. (2019, May 17). *How to do ego work*. The Holistic Psychologist. https://theholisticpsychologist.com/how-to-do-ego-work/

Nall, R. (2019, April 1). *What are the benefits of sunlight?* (T. J. Legg, Ed.). Healthline. https://www.healthline.com/health/depression/benefits-sunlight#benefits

Nash, J. (2022, June 19). *How to practice visualization meditation: 3 best scripts* (T. Sauber Millacci, Ed.). Positive Psychology. https://positivepsychology.com/visualization-meditation/

Nicotera, L. (n.d.). *The healing power of your thoughts and feelings*. The Ultra-Wellness Center. Retrieved November 29, 2022, from https://www.ultrawellnesscenter.com/2017/11/09/healing-power-thoughts-feelings/

Niemiec, R. (2016, April 25). *A mindful pause to change your day*. VIA Institute on Character. https://www.viacharacter.org/topics/articles/a-mindful-pause-to-change-your-day#:~:text=How%20to%20Do%20a%20Mindful

Northwestern Medicine. (2020, October). *5 things you never knew about fear*. https://www.nm.org/healthbeat/healthy-tips/emotional-health/5-things-you-never-knew-about-fear#:~:text=Fear%20is%20Physical&text=Stress%20hormones%20like%20cortisol%20and

Nunez, K. (2020a, August 10). *The benefits of progressive muscle relaxation and how to do it* (G. Minnis, Ed.). Healthline. https://www.healthline.com/health/progressive-muscle-relaxation

Nunez, K. (2020b, September 10). *The benefits of guided imagery and how to do it* (A. Klein, Ed.). Healthline. https://www.healthline.com/health/guided-imagery

Nunez, K. (2021, February 1). *What are the advantages of nose breathing vs. mouth breathing?* (C. T. Chavoustie, Ed.). Healthline. https://www.healthline.com/health/nose-breathing

Orion Philosophy. (2019, September 11). *What is Stoicism? A definition and three Stoic practices to start you off*. Medium. https://medium.com/@orion_philosophy/what-is-stoicism-a-definition-3-stoic-practices-to-start-you-off-139aef5248c3

Othership. (2021, August 19). *15 breathwork benefits: The science behind breathing practices*. (2021, August 19). Othership. https://www.othership.us/resources/breathwork-benefits

Owens, A. (2021, September 23). *Oxytocin*. Psycom. https://www.psycom.net/oxytocin

Parrott, J., & Goldie, J. (2019). *Best positive affirmations for anxiety relief: Reduce anxiety with affirmations*. National Road Safety Partnership Program. https://www.nrspp.org.au/resources/best-positive-affirmations-for-anxiety-relief/#:~:text=Simply-positive-affirmations-for-anxiety-a-soothing-and-calming-effect

Peripheral nervous system (PNS). (2022, May 25). Cleveland Clinic. https://my.clevelandclinic.org/health/body/23123-peripheral-nervous-system-pns#:~:text=Your%20peripheral%20nervous%20system%20(PNS)%20is%20that%20part%20of%20your

Pink Heart Healing. (2020). *What is creative visualization?* [Video]. YouTube. https://www.youtube.com/watch?v=zDAif7IjiO8

Psychogenic pain is real pain: Causes and treatments. (2017, March 20). Dignity Health. https://www.dignityhealth.org/articles/psychogenic-pain-is-real-pain-causes-and-treatments

Ray, A. (2010). *Om chanting and meditation.* In www.goodreads.com. Inner Light Publishers. https://www.goodreads.com/work/quotes/13887075

Raypole, C. (2020, May 28). *5 visualization techniques to add to your meditation practice* (T. J. Legg, Ed.). Healthline. https://www.healthline.com/health/visualization-meditation#guided-imagery

Raypole, C. (2021, January 8). *10 tips to take charge of your mindset and control your thoughts* (T. J. Legg, Ed.). Healthline. https://www.healthline.com/health/mental-health/how-to-control-your-mind#stress-management

Rodolfo, K. (2000, January 3). What is homeostasis? *Scientific American.* https://www.scientificamerican.com/article/what-is-homeostasis/

Rollo, N. (n.d.). *Square breathing: How to reduce stress through breathwork.* ZenCare. https://blog.zencare.co/square-breathing/

Roncero, A. (2021, August 3). *What is an existential crisis, and how do you overcome it?* BetterUp. https://www.betterup.com/blog/what-is-an-existential-crisis

Rosen, N. (Ed.). (2020, September 29). *How depression affects your immune system.* DispatchHealth. https://www.dispatchhealth.com/blog/how-depression-affects-your-immune-system/#:~:text=We

Rosenberg, J. (2017, November 11). The effects of chronic fear on a person's health. *The American Journal of Managed Care.* https://www.ajmc.com/view/the-effects-of-chronic-fear-on-a-persons-health

Saling, J. (2022, February 8). *What Is the placebo effect?* (C. DerSarkissian, Ed.). WebMD. https://www.webmd.com/pain-management/what-is-the-placebo-effect

Sarmah, A. (n.d.). *What is subconscious mind? Functions & parts of the subconscious mind.* MindWiper. Retrieved December 7, 2022, from https://mindwiper.com/what-is-subconscious-mind/

Saunders, J. L. (2022). Stoicism. In *Encyclopedia Britannica.* https://www.britannica.com/topic/Stoicism

Sauter, S., Murphy, L., Colligan, M., Swanson, N., Hurrell, Jr., J., Scharf, Jr., F., Sinclair, R., Grubb, P., Goldenhar, L., Alterman, T., Johnston, J., Hamilton, A., & Tisdale, J. (1999). *Stress...At work. Stress at Work, Publication no. 99-101.* Centers for Disease Control and Prevention. https://doi.org/10.26616/nioshpub99101

Scott, E. (2021, September 13). *Body scan meditation: Release tension with this targeted meditation technique* (M. Monahan, Ed.). Verywell Mind. https://www.verywellmind.com/body-scan-meditation-why-and-how-3144782

Sensory exercises. (2022, April). Sense. https://www.sense.org.uk/information-and-advice/for-professionals/sense-active-for-professionals/sensory-exercises/

Shah, S. (n.d.). *What is ego? 5 simple yet powerful ways to transcend the ego for good.* Art of Living. Retrieved December 9, 2022, from https://www.artofliving.org/us-en/what-is-ego-5-simple-yet-powerful-ways-to-transcend-the-ego-for-good

Shaver, R. (2019). Egoism. In E. N. Zalta (Ed.), *The Stanford Encyclopedia of Philosophy* (Winter 2021 Edition). https://plato.stanford.edu/archives/win2021/entries/egoism/

Sites, B., & Davis, T. (n.d.). *Positive affirmations: Definition, examples, and exercises.* Berkeley Well-Being Institute. Retrieved December 11, 2022, from https://www.berkeleywellbeing.com/positive-affirmations.html

Smith, A. J. (2021, November 8). *Gratitude - A mental health game changer.* Anxiety and Depression Association of America. https://adaa.org/learn-from-us/from-the-experts/blog-posts/consumer/gratitude-mental-health-game-changer

Smyth, J. M., Johnson, J. A., Auer, B. J., Lehman, E., Talamo, G., & Sciamanna, C. N. (2018). Online Positive Affect Journaling in the Improvement of Mental Distress and Well-Being in General medical patients with elevated anxiety symptoms: A preliminary randomized controlled trial. *JMIR Mental Health,* 5(4), e11290. PubMed Central. https://doi.org/10.2196/11290

Sörqvist, P. (2016). Grand challenges in environmental psychology. *Frontiers in Psychology,* 7(583). https://doi.org/10.3389/fpsyg.2016.00583

REFERENCES | 167

Spine Institute of North America. (n.d.). *5 positive affirmations for those recovering from joint pain*. Retrieved December 11, 2022, from https://spineina.com/blog/5-positive-affirmations-for-those-recovering-from-joint-pain/#:~:text=Research-shows-that-positive-thinking-our-experiences-and-changing-habits

Stanborough, R. J. (2019, October 15). *Benefits of reading books: How it can positively affect your life* (H. Moawad, Ed.). Healthline. https://www.healthline.com/health/benefits-of-reading-books

Star, K. (2022, March 10). *Using visualization to reduce anxiety symptoms* (M. Monahan, Ed.). VerywellMind. https://www.verywellmind.com/visualization-for-relaxation-2584112

Subconscious. (n.d.). *Merriam-Webster*. https://www.merriam-webster.com/dictionary/subconscious

Surrenda, D. (2012). The purpose of yoga. *New York Times*. https://www.nytimes.com/roomfordebate/2012/01/12/is-yoga-for-narcissists/the-purpose-of-yoga

Take a deep breath. (2012, August 10). The American Institute of Stress. https://www.stress.org/take-a-deep-breath

The birth of physics – The Ancient Greeks to the Renaissance. (2012, December 2). Physics 139. https://blogs.umass.edu/p139ell/

The meditations of Marcus Aurelius Antoninus (J. Jackson, Trans.). (1906). Oxford at the Clarendon Press. https://books.google.co.za/books?id=8msvRVmsO8EC&pg=PA2&source=kp_read_button&hl=en&redir_esc=y#v=onepage&q&f=false

The power of your subconscious mind. (n.d.). Brian Tracy International. https://www.briantracy.com/blog/personal-success/understanding-your-subconscious-mind/

Therapy for You. (2020, March 4). *21 top tips on practicing mindfulness for beginners*. (2020, March 4). Therapy for You. https://www.therapyforyou.co.uk/post/practicing-mindfulness-for-beginners

The visualization definition and how It transforms your life. (2022, July 11). BetterHelp. https://www.betterhelp.com/advice/visualization/the-visualization-definition-and-how-it-transforms-your-life/

Trauma. (n.d.). American Psychological Association. Retrieved December 11, 2022, from https://www.apa.org/topics/trauma#:~:text=Trauma%20is%20an%20emotional%20response

Tucker, A. (2020, December 23). *How to start a mindful journaling practice*. Mindful. https://www.mindful.org/how-to-start-a-mindful-journaling-practice/#:~:text=Mindful%20journaling%20allows%20the%20space

Tucker, I. (2016, February 15). All in the mind? How research is proving the true healing power of the placebo. *The Guardian*. https://www.theguardian.com/science/2016/feb/15/jo-marchant-mind-body-health-medicine-science

Upham, B. (2021, November 12). *Deep breathing: A complete guide to the relaxation technique*. Everyday Health. https://www.everydayhealth.com/wellness/deep-breathing/

Visualization and guided imagery techniques for stress reduction. (n.d.). Mental-Help. Retrieved December 11, 2022, from https://www.mental-help.net/stress/visualization-and-guided%20-imagery-techniques-for-stress-reduction/#:~:text=Take%2%200a%20few%20slow%20and,sitting%20on%20a%20favorite%20%20chair

von Bernhardi, R., Bernhardi, L. E., & Eugenín, J. (2017). What is neural plasticity? *Advances in Experimental Medicine and Biology*, 1015, 1–15. Pub Med. https://doi.org/10.1007/978-3-319-62817-2_1

Voss, M. W., Savoie-Roskos, M., Coombs, C., Murza, G., Nelson, C., & Withers, E. (n.d.). *Exercise and chronic pain*. Utah State University. Retrieved December 12, 2022, from https://extension.usu.edu/heart/research/exercise-and-chronic-pain#:~:text=Individuals-suffering-from-chronic-pain-pain-sensitivity-C-and-reducing-inflammation

Waxenbaum, J. A., Reddy, V., & Varacallo, M. (2020, August 10). *Anatomy, Autonomic Nervous System*. PubMed; StatPearls Publishing. https://www.ncbi.nlm.nih.gov/books/NBK539845/#:~:text=The%20autonomic%20nervous%20system%20is

"We give life to what we give energy to" - Manifesting. (n.d.). Live to Be a Legend. Retrieved November 29, 2022, from https://livetobealegend.com/manifesting/transformational-quotes/#:~:text=How%20we%20choose%20to%20spend

What do we mean by inner and outer worlds? (n.d.). The Good Society. Retrieved December 7, 2022, from https://thegoodsociety.gov.au/guidebook/years-10-12-guidebook/chapter-2---influences/inner--outer-worlds/what-do-we-mean-by-inner-and-outer-worlds

What is creative visualization? (2022, December 8). BetterHelp. https://www.betterhelp.com/advice/visualization/what-is-creative-visualization/

What is mindfulness? (2020, July 8). Mindful. https://www.mindful.org/what-is-mindfulness/

Winne, P. H., & Azevedo, R. (2014). Metacognition. *The Cambridge Handbook of the Learning Sciences*, 63–87. American Psychological Assocication PsycNet. https://doi.org/10.1017/cbo9781139519526.006

Winston, D. (n.d.). *Mindful breathing*. Greater Good in Action; University of California, Berkeley. https://ggia.berkeley.edu/practice/mindful_breathing#:~:text=Sometimes%2C%20especially%20when%20trying%20to

Zundel, C. G. (n.d.). Air pollution harms the brain and mental health, too, a large-scale analysis shows. *News 24*. Retrieved December 9, 2022, from https://www.news24.com/life/wellness/mind/air-pollution-harms-the-brain-and-mental-health-too-a-large-scale-analysis-shows-20221127

Printed in Great Britain
by Amazon